Adjunct Interventions to Cognitive Behavioral Therapy for Insomnia

Editor

JOSHUA HYONG-JIN CHO

SLEEP MEDICINE CLINICS

www.sleep.theclinics.com

March 2023 • Volume 18 • Number 1

ELSEVIER

1600 John F. Kennedy Boulevard • Suite 1800 • Philadelphia, Pennsylvania, 19103-2899

http://www.theclinics.com

SLEEP MEDICINE CLINICS Volume 18, Number 1
March 2023, ISSN 1556-407X, ISBN-13: 978-0-323-93965-2

Editor: Joanna Collett
Developmental Editor: Axell Ivan Jade M. Purificacion

Sleep Medicine Clinics (ISSN 1556-407X) is published quarterly by Elsevier Inc., 360 Park Avenue South, New York, NY 10010-1710. Months of issue are March, June, September and December. Business and Editorial Offices: 1600 John F. Kennedy Blvd., Ste. 1800, Philadelphia, PA 19103-2899. Customer Service Office: 3251 Riverport Lane, Maryland Heights, MO 63043. Periodicals postage paid at New York, NY and additional mailing offices. Subscription prices are $243.00 per year (US individuals), $100.00 (US and Canadian students), $612.00 (US institutions), $283.00 (Canadian individuals), $278.00 (international individuals) $135.00 (International students), $692.00 (Canadian and International institutions). Foreign air speed delivery is included in all *Clinics* subscription prices. All prices are subject to change without notice. **POSTMASTER:** Send change of address to *Sleep Medicine Clinics*, Elsevier Health Sciences Division, Subscription Customer Service, 3251 Riverport Lane, Maryland Heights, MO 63043. Customer Service: **Tel: 1-800-654-2452 (U.S. and Canada); 314-447-8871 (outside U.S. and Canada). Fax: 314-447-8029. E-mail: journalscustomerservice-usa@elsevier.com (for print support); journalsonline-support-usa@elsevier.com (for online support).**

Reprints. For copies of 100 or more of articles in this publication, please contact the Commercial Reprints Department, Elsevier Inc., 360 Park Avenue South, New York, NY 10010-1710. Tel.: 212-633-3874; Fax: 212-633-3820; E-mail: reprints@elsevier.com.

Sleep Medicine Clinics is covered in *MEDLINE/PubMed (Index Medicus)*.

SLEEP MEDICINE CLINICS

FORTHCOMING ISSUES

June 2023
Pediatric Sleep Clinics
Haviva Veler, *Editor*

September 2023
Advances in Technology for the Sleep Field
Steven Holfinger, *Editor*

December 2023
Sleep in Women
Monica Andersen, *Editor*

RECENT ISSUES

December 2022
A review of PAP therapy for the treatment of OSA
Matthew R. Ebben, *Editor*

September 2022
Commemorative Issue: 15 Years of the Sleep Medicine Clinics Part 2: Medication and Treatment Effect on Sleep Disorders
Ana C. Krieger and Teofilo Lee-Chiong, *Editors*

June 2022
Commemorative Issue: 15 Years of the Sleep Medicine Clinics Part 1: Sleep and Sleep Disorders
Ana C. Krieger and Teofilo Lee-Chiong, *Editors*

SERIES OF RELATED INTEREST

Psychiatric Clinics
https://www.psych.theclinics.com/
Medical Clinics
https://www.medical.theclinics.com/

THE CLINICS ARE AVAILABLE ONLINE!
Access your subscription at:
www.theclinics.com

Contributors

CONSULTING EDITORS

TEOFILO LEE-CHIONG Jr, MD
Professor of Medicine, National Jewish Health, Professor of Medicine, University of Colorado, Denver, Colorado, USA; Chief Medical Liaison, Philips Respironics, Murrysville, Pennsylvania, USA

ANA C. KRIEGER, MD, MPH, FCCP, FAASM
Chief, Division of Sleep Neurology, Medical, Director, Weill Cornell Center for Sleep Medicine, Professor of Clinical Medicine, Professor of Medicine in Neurology and Genetic Medicine, Weill Cornell Medical College, Cornell University, New York, New York, USA

EDITOR

JOSHUA HYONG-JIN CHO, MD, PhD
Professor, Director, UCLA Insomnia Clinic, Faculty, Cousins Center for Psychoneuroimmunology, Department of

Psychiatry & Biobehavioral Sciences, David Geffen School of Medicine at UCLA, Los Angeles, California, USA

AUTHORS

PAMELA ALFONSO-MILLER, MD
Northumbria Sleep Research, Northumbria University, Newcastle, United Kingdom

PAUL BARKOPOULOS, MD, MPH
Clinical Professor, Department of Psychiatry and Biobehavioral Sciences, UCLA David Geffen School of Medicine, UCLA Insomnia Clinic, Cousins Center for Psychoneuroimmunology, University of California, Los Angeles, Cedars Sinai Medical Center, Los Angeles, California, USA

CÉLYNE H. BASTIEN, PhD
École de Psychologie, Pavillon Félix-Antoine-Savard, Université Laval, Québec (Québec), Canada

DARAH-BREE BENSEN-BOAKES, B.Psyc (Hons)
Flinders Health and Medical Research Institute: Sleep Health, Flinders University, Adelaide, South Australia

TANECIA BLUE, PhD, ABPP, VA
Pacific Islands Healthcare System, Honolulu, Hawaii, USA

JOSHUA HYONG-JIN CHO, MD, PhD
Clinical Professor, Director, Department of Psychiatry and Biobehavioral Sciences, UCLA David Geffen School of Medicine, UCLA Insomnia Clinic, Cousins Center for Psychoneuroimmunology, University of California, Los Angeles, Los Angeles, California, USA

JASON GORDON ELLIS, PhD
Northumbria Sleep Research, Faculty of Health and Life Sciences, Northumbria University, Newcastle, United Kingdom; Department of Physical Education and Sport Sciences, University of Limerick, Sreelane, Castletroy, Co. Limerick, Ireland

SHEILA. N. GARLAND, PhD
Department of Psychology, Faculty of Science, Memorial University, Discipline of Oncology,

Faculty of Medicine, Memorial University, St John's, Newfoundland, Canada

MARKUS JANSSON-FRÖJMARK, PhD
Department of Clinical Neuroscience, Centre for Psychiatry Research, Karolinska Institutet, Stockholm Health Care Services, Competence Center for Psychotherapy Research and Education, Stockholm, Sweden

DAVID A. KALMBACH, PhD
Assistant Scientist, Thomas Roth Sleep Disorders Center, Henry Ford Health System, Assistant Professor, Department of Pulmonary and Critical Care and Sleep Medicine, Wayne State University School of Medicine, Detroit, Michigan, USA

STEPHANIE KREMER, PsyD
Assistant Clinical Professor, Department of Psychiatry and Biobehavioral Sciences, UCLA David Geffen School of Medicine, UCLA Insomnia Clinic, Cousins Center for Psychoneuroimmunology, Los Angeles, California, USA

SAMLAU KUTANA, BA
Department of Psychology, Faculty of Science, Memorial University, St John's, Newfoundland, Canada

LEON LACK, PhD
Flinders Health and Medical Research Institute: Sleep Health, Flinders University, Adelaide, South Australia

NICOLE LOVATO, PhD
Flinders Health and Medical Research Institute: Sleep Health, Flinders University, Adelaide, South Australia

JUN J. MAO, MD, MSCE
Department of Medicine, Memorial Sloan Kettering Cancer Center, New York, New York, USA

JENNIFER L. MARTIN, PhD
VA Greater Los Angeles Healthcare System, Geriatric Research, Education, and Clinical Center, North Hills, Department of Medicine, UCLA David Geffen School of Medicine, University of California, Los Angeles, Los Angeles, California, USA

SARAH KATE MCGOWAN, PhD
Department of Psychiatry and Biobehavioral Sciences, UCLA David Geffen School of Medicine, University of California, Los Angeles, Department of Mental Health, VA Greater Los Angeles Healthcare System, Los Angeles, California, USA

ROBERT MEADOWS, PhD
Department of Sociology, University of Surrey, Guildford, United Kingdom

TARA MURALI, B.Psyc (Hons)
College of Education, Psychology and Social Work, Flinders University, Adelaide, South Australia

ANNIKA NORELL-CLARKE, PhD
Karlstad University, Karlstad, Sweden; Department of Law, Psychology and Social Work, Örebro University, Örebro, Sweden; Faculty of Health Sciences, Kristianstad University, Kristianstad, Sweden

JASON C. ONG, PhD
Adjunct Associate Professor, Department of Neurology, Center for Circadian and Sleep Medicine, Northwestern University Feinberg School of Medicine, Chicago, Illinois, USA; Director, Behavioral Sleep Medicine, Nox Health, Suwanee, Georgia, USA

GISELLE SOARES PASSOS, PhD
Professor, Health Sciences Unit, Universidade Federal de Jataí, Jataí, GO, Brazil

GRETA B. RAGLAN, PhD
Assistant Professor, Department of Psychiatry, University of Michigan, Ann Arbor, Michigan, USA

KATHRYN S. SALDAÑA, PhD
Department of Mental Health, VA Greater Los Angeles Healthcare System, Los Angeles, California, USA

CHRISTINA SANDLUND, PhD
Department of Neurobiology, Care Sciences and Society, Academic Primary Health Care Centre, Karolinska Institutet, Stockholm, Sweden

MARCOS GONÇALVES SANTANA, PhD
Professor, Health Sciences Unit, Universidade
Federal de Jataí, Jataí, GO, Brazil

HANNAH SCOTT, PhD
Flinders Health and Medical Research Institute:
Sleep Health, Flinders University, Adelaide,
South Australia

LESLIE M. SWANSON, PhD
Associate Professor, Department of
Psychiatry, University of Michigan, Ann Arbor,
Michigan, USA

JEFFREY YOUNG, PhD, CBSM, DBSM
Associate Clinical Professor, UCLA David
Geffen School of Medicine, Semel Institute of
Neuroscience and Human Behavior, UCLA
Insomnia Clinic, Los Angeles, California, USA

SHAWN D. YOUNGSTEDT, PhD
Professor, Edson College of Nursing and
Health Innovation, Arizona State University,
Phoenix, Arizona, USA

Contents

Preface: Adjunct Interventions to Cognitive Behavioral Therapy for Insomnia   xiii

Joshua Hyong-Jin Cho

Partner Alliance to Enhance Efficacy and Adherence of CBT-I   1

Jason Gordon Ellis, Robert Meadows, Pamela Alfonso-Miller, and Célyne H. Bastien

> Cognitive behavioral therapy for insomnia (CBT-I) is now widely recognized as the first-line management strategy for insomnia, both for insomnia in its "pure" form, and when comorbid with a physical or psychological illness. However, there is a definite need to develop and test both alternative and adjunct interventions to CBT-I, before implementing them into routine practice. The aim of this article is to provide a narrative review of the literature with regard to what is known about the influence of partners on sleep, insomnia, and its management.

Paradoxic Intention as an Adjunct Treatment to Cognitive Behavioral Therapy for Insomnia   9

Markus Jansson-Fröjmark, Christina Sandlund, and Annika Norell-Clarke

> Paradoxic intention (PI) was one of the first psychological interventions for insomnia. Historically, PI has been incorporated in cognitive behavioral therapy for insomnia (CBT-I) or delivered as a sole intervention for insomnia. PI instructions have varied over the years, but a common denominator is the instruction to try to stay awake in bed for as long as possible. This article reviews and discuss treatment rationales and theoretic frameworks for PI, the current evidence base for PI, its clinical relevance, and considerations needed when PI is used as an adjunct treatment to CBT-I, or as a second-line intervention for insomnia.

Circadian Interventions as Adjunctive Therapies to Cognitive-Behavioral Therapy for Insomnia   21

Leslie M. Swanson and Greta B. Raglan

> The circadian system plays a key role in the sleep-wake cycle. A mismatch between the behavioral timing of sleep and the circadian timing of sleepiness/alertness can contribute to insomnia. Patients who report primarily difficulty falling asleep or early morning awakenings may benefit from circadian interventions administered adjunctively to cognitive-behavioral therapy for insomnia. Specific circadian interventions that clinicians may consider include bright light therapy, scheduled dim light, blue-blocking glasses, and melatonin. Implementation of these interventions differs depending on the patient's insomnia subtype. Further, careful attention must be paid to the timing of these interventions to ensure they are administered correctly.

Behavioral Activation as an Adjunct Treatment to CBT-I   31

Jeffrey Young

> Behavioral activation (BA) has long been long understood to be a particularly effective treatment for depression. Elements of BA are also to be found in components of insomnia treatment such as sleep restriction, stimulus control, and the setting of a morning routine. Although little research exists that examines the independent contribution of BA to the treatment of insomnia, it is reasonable to apportion some of the effect of cognitive-behavioral treatment of insomnia (CBT-I) to the implementation of BA whether that implementation is simply incidental to standard practice or more extensively deployed.

Exercise as an Adjunct Treatment to Cognitive Behavior Therapy for Insomnia   39

Giselle Soares Passos, Shawn D. Youngstedt, and Marcos Gonçalves Santana

> The question that guided this review is whether exercise can add to the improvements in insomnia in patients treated with cognitive behavioral therapy for insomnia (CBT-I). CBT-I has long been recommended as the first-line treatment of chronic insomnia. However, CBT-I is not effective for as many as 30% to 40% of patients with insomnia. There is accumulating evidence for positive effects on insomnia following acute and chronic exercise. However, to the best of our knowledge, the effects of CBT-I combined with exercise have not been explored in clinical trials. In this article, we develop a rationale for combining CBT-I with exercise.

Wearable Device-Delivered Intensive Sleep Retraining as an Adjunctive Treatment to Kickstart Cognitive-Behavioral Therapy for Insomnia   49

Darah-Bree Bensen-Boakes, Tara Murali, Nicole Lovato, Leon Lack, and Hannah Scott

> Intensive Sleep Retraining is a behavioral treatment for sleep onset insomnia that produces substantial benefits in symptoms after a single treatment session. This technique involves falling asleep and waking up shortly afterward repeatedly: a process that is thought to retrain people to fall asleep quickly when attempting sleep. Although originally confined to the sleep laboratory, recent technological developments mean that this technique is feasible to self-administer at home. With multiple randomised controlled trials required to confirm its efficacy, Intensive Sleep Retraining may serve as an adjunctive treatment to cognitive-behavioral therapy for insomnia, improving short-term efficacy by kick-starting treatment gains.

Mindfulness as an Adjunct or Alternative to CBT-I   59

Jason C. Ong and David A. Kalmbach

> Mindfulness-based interventions (MBIs) are programs that teach mindfulness concepts through guided meditation and self-regulation practices. MBIs have been found to improve sleep and reduce cognitive arousal, which are central to the development and perpetuation of insomnia. In this article, we review theoretic frameworks and clinical trial effectiveness data supporting MBIs for insomnia. Based on this review, we provide suggestions for using MBIs as an adjunct or alternative treatment option to CBT-I with regard to how, when, and for whom. We conclude with an agenda for future directions that can clarify the use of mindfulness as a treatment option for insomnia.

Acceptance and Commitment Therapy as an Adjunct or Alternative Treatment to Cognitive Behavioral Therapy for Insomnia   73

Kathryn S. Saldaña, Sarah Kate McGowan, and Jennifer L. Martin

> Although cognitive behavioral therapy for insomnia (CBT-I) is an effective treatment of insomnia, difficulties exist with adherence to recommendations and premature discontinuation of treatment does occur. The current article aims to review existing research on acceptance and commitment therapy (ACT)-based interventions, demonstrate differences and similarities between ACT for insomnia and CBT-I, and describe treatment components and mechanisms of ACT that can be used to treat insomnia disorder.

Biofeedback as an Adjunct or Alternative Intervention to Cognitive Behavioral Therapy for Insomnia   85

Stephanie Kremer and Tanecia Blue

> Insomnia is highly prevalent and comorbid with many disorders. However, insomnia is underdiagnosed and undertreated in many populations. Cognitive behavioral

therapy for insomnia (CBT-I) is not appropriate or sufficient for some individuals. Biofeedback has demonstrated efficacy in a range of disorders, including insomnia. The authors discuss the history and rationale for the use of biofeedback in the treatment of insomnia and other comorbid disorders. The article also presents current research on biofeedback for insomnia and comorbid disorders with recommendations for using biofeedback as an adjunct or alternative intervention to CBT-I.

Hypnotic Medications as an Adjunct Treatment to Cognitive Behavioral Therapy for Insomnia   95

Paul Barkopoulos and Joshua Hyong-Jin Cho

Cognitive behavioral therapy for insomnia (CBT-I) is the universally recommended treatment of choice for insomnia disorder based on its safety and posttreatment durability of benefit. However, CBT-I does not help all patients achieve remission. The second most evidence-based treatment, hypnotic pharmacotherapy (PCT), does not resolve perpetuating factors of insomnia, resulting in potential waning of benefit and dependence. This article presents a rationale that supports consideration of hypnotic augmentation of CBT-I (COMB), along with a review of select randomized controlled trials relevant to clinical decision-making.

Acupuncture as an Adjunct Treatment to Cognitive-Behavioral Therapy for Insomnia   113

Samlau Kutana, Jun J. Mao, and Sheila.N. Garland

Cognitive-behavioral therapy for insomnia (CBT-I) is the main recommended treatment for patients presenting with insomnia; however, the treatment is not equally effective for all, and several factors can contribute to a diminished treatment response. The rationale for combining CBT-I treatment with acupuncture is explored, and evidence supporting its use in treating insomnia and related comorbidities is discussed. Practical, regulatory, and logistical issues with implementing a combined treatment are examined, and future directions for research are made. Growing evidence supports the effectiveness of acupuncture in treating insomnia and comorbid conditions, and warrants further investigation of acupuncture as an adjunct to CBT-I.

Preface

Adjunct Interventions to Cognitive Behavioral Therapy for Insomnia

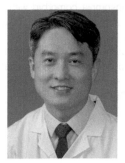

Joshua Hyong-Jin Cho, MD, PhD
Editor

Cognitive Behavioral Therapy for Insomnia (CBT-I) has been consistently demonstrated to be an efficacious treatment of insomnia[1] and is widely acknowledged as the first-line treatment for insomnia.[2,3] However, because CBT-I essentially consists of cognitive restructuring and behavior modification that require patient engagement and their active participation, it has inherent limitations. First, suboptimal adherence to CBT-I components is a known limitation and reduces its impact.[4] Second, a considerable proportion of patients drop out, with attrition rates in sleep clinics ranging from 10% to 40%.[5] Third, approximately 40% of patients that participate in randomized controlled trials of CBT-I achieves remission, which is a respectable success rate for a mental/behavioral health condition but still highly unsatisfying.[6,7] Thus, adjunct interventions that overcome such limitations of CBT-I would be of paramount importance in clinical practice. This issue reviews behavioral (B), pharmacologic (P), and other (O) interventions that may complement and/or serve as an alternative option to CBT-I.

Most interventions addressed in this issue serve as adjunct treatments to CBT-I, including paradoxical intention (B), circadian rhythm regulation (B and P), behavioral activation (B), exercise (B), intense sleep retraining (B), and acupuncture (O). Although hypnotic medications (P) are often used as an alternative treatment to CBT-I in clinical practice, given the clear superiority of CBT-I especially in the long term, they are reviewed in this issue as an adjunct treatment to CBT-I. Two interventions may serve as both adjunct and alternative treatments to CBT-I: mindfulness (B) and acceptance and commitment therapy (B). Last, partner alliance (O) is not a treatment per se but is addressed in this issue as a means to complement and enhance CBT-I.

Out of the 11 interventions described in the issue, four are supported by a reasonable amount of largely consistent evidence: mindfulness, circadian rhythm regulation, exercise, and acupuncture. Several clinical trials exist that tested hypnotic medications as an adjunct treatment to CBT-I; however, the data are complex, requiring a careful interpretation. The other interventions reviewed in the issue have less-extensive or less-consistent evidence, while they are all based on robust theoretical rationales: partner alliance, paradoxical intention, behavioral activation, intense sleep retraining, acceptance and commitment therapy, and biofeedback.

Joshua Hyong-Jin Cho, MD, PhD
UCLA Insomnia Clinic
Department of Psychiatry and Biobehavioral Sciences
David Geffen School of Medicine at UCLA
300 UCLA Medical Plaza, Suite 3200A
Los Angeles, CA 90095, USA

E-mail address:
hjcho@mednet.ucla.edu

Sleep Med Clin 18 (2023) xiii–xiv
https://doi.org/10.1016/j.jsmc.2022.12.001
1556-407X/23/© 2022 Published by Elsevier Inc.

REFERENCES

1. Trauer JM, Qian MY, Doyle JS, et al. Cognitive behavioral therapy for chronic insomnia: a systematic review and meta-analysis. Ann Intern Med 2015; 163(3):191–204.
2. Morgenthaler T, Kramer M, Alessi C, et al. Practice parameters for the psychological and behavioral treatment of insomnia: an update. An American Academy of Sleep Medicine Report. Sleep 2006;29(11):1415–9.
3. Qaseem A, Kansagara D, Forciea MA, et al, Clinical Guidelines Committee of the American College of P. Management of chronic insomnia disorder in adults: a clinical practice guideline from the American College of Physicians. Ann Intern Med 2016;165(2):125–33.
4. Matthews EE, Arnedt JT, McCarthy MS, et al. Adherence to cognitive behavioral therapy for insomnia: a systematic review. Sleep Med Rev 2013;17(6):453–64.
5. Ong JC, Kuo TF, Manber R. Who is at risk for dropout from group cognitive-behavior therapy for insomnia? J Psychosom Res 2008;64(4):419–25.
6. Wu JQ, Appleman ER, Salazar RD, et al. Cognitive behavioral therapy for insomnia comorbid with psychiatric and medical conditions: a meta-analysis. JAMA Intern Med 2015;175(9):1461–72.
7. Morin CM, Vallieres A, Guay B, et al. Cognitive behavioral therapy, singly and combined with medication, for persistent insomnia: a randomized controlled trial. JAMA 2009;301(19):2005–15.

Partner Alliance to Enhance Efficacy and Adherence of CBT-I

Jason Gordon Ellis, PhD[a,b,*], Robert Meadows, PhD[c],
Pamela Alfonso-Miller, MD[a], Célyne H. Bastien, PhD[d]

KEYWORDS

• CBT-I • Partners • Adjunct • Social support • Therapy

KEY POINTS

• Although cognitive behavioral therapy for insomnia (CBT-I) is largely effective and efficacious, it is not without its challenges.
• Future research could look to socio-ecological dimensions, as a starting point, when creating new adjunct therapies for CBT-I.
• Very limited research have been undertaken on understanding the relationship between insomnia and being in a relationship, beyond the burden of caregiving.
• Partners can influence uptake and engagement with CBT-I.
• Including partners in CBT-I may be a beneficial step in increasing adherence and treatment outcomes but more research is needed.

INTRODUCTION

Despite cognitive behavioral therapy for insomnia (CBT-I) existing, being studied, and used for decades, only relatively recently has it been advocated as the first-line treatment.[1,2] The time taken to accumulate compelling amounts of robust CBT-I study data (including health economic data[3]), alongside increasing awareness of the limitations of existing treatments (eg, pharmacotherapy, sleep hygiene as a monotherapy[4]), presumably underscore the lag in time between its development and it being advocated so widely. That said, and despite the thousands of published CBT-I studies in existence, CBT-I is not without its challenges. Although at a cohort level its efficacy and effectiveness are well established, approximately 30% to 50% of individuals do not achieve

"remission" following CBT-I,[5,6] although this can be influenced by how remission is measured.[7] Further, several issues have been highlighted concerning uptake (particularly for digital CBT-I), attrition, and adherence.[8–12] The reasons for these challenges are likely multifactorial; however, one area gaining traction is the impact of sociocultural factors on overall sleep health.[13] Within this framework, although the individual is still acknowledged as being a "central agent" in understanding and managing their own sleep health (microsystem), other factors can influence an individual's sleep or perception thereof; from a mesosystem level perspective (eg, family, work, culture) or a macrosystem level perspective (eg, society, government, technology, policy).

Although the socio-ecological model has not been applied specifically within the context of

a Northumbria Sleep Research, Northumbria University, 129 NB408 Northumberland Building, Newcastle, NE1 8ST, United Kingdom; b Department of Physical Education and Sport Sciences, University of Limerick, Sreelane, Castletroy, Co. Limerick, V94 T9PX, Ireland; c Department of Sociology, University of Surrey, 15 AD 03, GU2 7XH, United Kingdom; d École de Psychologie, Pavillon Félix-Antoine-Savard, Université Laval, 2325, Rue des Bibliothèques, Local 1012, Québec (Québec) G1V 0A6, Canada
* Corresponding author.
E-mail address: Jason.ellis@northumbria.ac.uk

Sleep Med Clin 18 (2023) 1–7
https://doi.org/10.1016/j.jsmc.2022.09.005
1556-407X/23/Crown Copyright © 2022 Published by Elsevier Inc. All rights reserved.

behavioral sleep medicine (BSM), several pertinent factors, from each level, have been independently explored as potential influencers on sleep health or vice versa. One such area is the role of family and in particular partners.[14] This is logical considering the dyadic nature of sleep for a significant proportion of the population and the potential influence one partner's sleep, in terms of quality, quantity, timing, and disordered status, could have on the others.[15,16] Although partners have been clearly demonstrated as influential in the area of help seeking behavior for individuals with sleep-related breathing disorders, its treatment using continuous positive airway pressure (CPAP), and adherence to CPAP,[17,18] their role in other sleep disorders, specifically insomnia is less clear.[19]

Understanding the Role of Partners in the Context of Insomnia:

Broadly, being divorced is associated with higher levels of sleep disturbance compared with being married and being happily married is associated with fewer sleep disturbances compared with being unhappy or discontent in the marriage.[20] Moreover, having a sleep disturbance has been shown to partially mediate the relationship between interpersonal violence and physical and mental health, suggesting a role for sleep in mitigating the psychological impact of this violence.[21,22] Although these studies reinforce the idea that sleep disturbances and partner status are associated, albeit in complex ways, the cross-sectional or retrospective nature of these designs preclude an understanding of how exactly these factors are related. Moreover, the term sleep disturbances could imply several dimensions of sleep health, not all of which may be related to insomnia per se.

The majority of research specific to partners and insomnia has focused on insomnia being a product of caregiving for a chronically ill partner, such as those with cancer, Alzheimer disease or Parkinson disease.[23-25] The findings from these studies all tend to agree that having a partner with a chronic illness is associated with poorer sleep in general and increased insomnia symptoms. Implied in this research is that these additional factors surrounding the relationship (eg, increased caregiving burden, the chronically ill partner's impaired sleep or daytime functioning, multiple losses surrounding the illness) cause and maintain the insomnia. Alternatively, several cross-sectional studies have demonstrated that having a partner with insomnia, after controlling for confounding factors on the relationship, such as health status, is associated with poorer mental and physical health, poorer mood, and more dissatisfaction in

the relationship.[26-28] Additionally, having insomnia has been associated with decreased libido, which may further exacerbate relationship difficulties.[29] Moreover, one longitudinal study found that having a partner with insomnia conferred an increased risk for incident heart disease in adult men, but not women, during a 4-year period, after controlling for several relevant variables.[30] One potential reason for this latter finding may be that the concordance in objective sleep, usually observed in normally sleeping couples, is also evident in insomnia. In other words, although normally sleeping couples tend to mirror each other's sleep in several ways, and this may also occur if one partner has insomnia. Evidence for this is limited but one study showed that a good sleeping partner was 1.25 times more likely to awaken in response to their partner (the one with insomnia) waking during the night.[31] Alternatively, the quality of the relationship may be itself a precipitant or perpetuating factor to the insomnia.[32] Certainly, in one study on relationship counseling with individuals with insomnia and relationship difficulties, increases in marital satisfaction reduced the risk of insomnia by up to 36% in male partners but not female partners.[33] Irrespective of the pathway, it seems that insomnia and being in a relationship are intimately tied phenomena.

Can Partners Influence Cognitive Behavioral Therapy For Insomnia?

From this existing evidence, although limited, it could be argued that while partners are likely to be affected by having a bed partner with insomnia, underscoring the need for treatment, they may also be influential in its treatment. For example, a few studies have shown that partner treatment preferences are an important determinate of a patients' choice when considering how they manage their insomnia.[34,35] Moreover, the provision of social support by partners has been highlighted as an important factor in adherence to CBT-I.[36,37] Further to treatment seeking behavior and social support, Rogojanski and colleagues[19] point to several other areas where partners may be helpful during the process of CBT-I. First, they suggest inviting the partner to the first session (ie, clinical interview assessment)—suggesting this could be beneficial in terms of orienting both the patient and the partner to the therapy itself and what it is likely to entail, creating "buy in" from both parties. This would also identify potential individual or dyadic barriers or misunderstandings about what is and what is not involved from the outset. They suggest this is also an opportunity to determine as to whether it would be beneficial to include the partner (subject to both parties agreeing) in further sessions. Within the components of CBT-I, several other areas whereby partners could add value are highlighted. For example, to promote adherence to the behavioral components or to assist with distraction away from sleep-related thoughts and preoccupations and catastrophic interpretations. Beyond the therapy itself, they also identify a role for partners in relapse prevention in terms of helping the patient identify and manage high-risk situations, which could lead to relapse, or reinstigating therapy if necessary. One of the main issues highlighted, however, is attempts to address a mismatch in chronotype, if it exists. Although not examined within the area of insomnia, per se, several studies have demonstrated that having a mismatch (ie, one partner being more morning oriented and the other being more evening oriented) is associated with higher levels of relationship conflict and dissatisfaction.[38–40] One suggested method to address this, although founded on clinical practice as opposed to research has been the introduction of "cuddle time."[41] This would suggest that if there were a discrepancy in the preferred timing of sleep, the partner who is more inclined to go to bed later still goes to bed with the partner who is more morning oriented but there is no intention to sleep, just be with the other person. It is also suggested that this method can be applied in the context of sleep restriction therapy when a later time to bed is prescribed.

Only one study to date, however, has specifically examined the broad potential role partners could play throughout the course of CBT-I.[42] In this study, 21 individuals who had completed CBT-I were interviewed about their experiences. Using a BSM-specific motivational interviewing technique,[43] participants were asked what factors they thought led to how well they engaged with CBT-I and what factors may have further improved their level of engagement. They were also asked what factors are likely to be important to maintaining any treatment gains they had made. Using a quantitative content analysis, units of analysis (sentences), which explicitly mentioned partners were coded in an open manifest approach and designated as either positive (eg, my partner stayed up with me until my prescribed time to bed) or negative (eg, my partner does not believe in these [talking] types of therapies). Although the number of positive statements made about partner support was associated with positive treatment outcomes, negative statements were unrelated to any treatment outcomes. The results from the interviews also identified three core areas where partners can influence CBT-I, positively or negatively, namely discussion from the partner, actions by the partner, or thoughts held by the partner (**Table 1**).

It was concluded that partners could potentially play a role in CBT-I, being somewhere on a continuum between partner-related therapeutic alliance (ie, providing support) to being unhelpful or even obstructive to the process. Interestingly another dimension involving partners was also identified during the interviews—partner reliance—although not explicitly termed that by the patients. Partner reliance was demonstrated in cases whereby the partner became a "gatekeeper" for managing elements of treatment, with examples including making sure the individual did not fall asleep on the sofa in the evening and being instructed to waking them if they did, being responsible for waking the individual up in the morning if they slept past their prescribed time to wake or stopping the individual from doing something that would go against sleep hygiene advice (eg, making coffee in the early evening).

How these findings translate into the routine practice of CBT-I is unknown; however, one ongoing trial examining how "partner-assisted" CBT-I compares to standard CBT-I may soon provide the answers.[44] In this case the "partner-assisted" adjuvant is aimed to address sleep as an issue, not the relationship, through increasing social support and positive reinforcement. This is to be achieved through educating the partner about all the concepts (including the provision of tailored handouts), engaging them in the decision-making process during therapy and actively involving them in the process by determining how they may assist.

Future Directions

One of the main challenges is that CBT-I is still not a standardized therapy in terms of its components, delivery modality, structure or level of therapist training. As such, comparisons between CBT-I trials, let alone CBT-I trials with partner inclusion (in whichever capacity), should be examined with a certain degree of caution.

Clearly, more research is needed in the area of the impact of partners on CBT-I before it is introduced into standard care as an adjunct. There are still significant gaps in the literature as to the impact of relationship functioning in insomnia, and vice versa, as well as the identification of areas whereby partners can affect treatment (both positively and negatively). One fruitful way forward would be to have naturalistic studies, which track both sleep and relationship functioning to determine the relative impact of each

Table 1
Partner-related factors that influence the course of cognitive behavioral therapy for insomnia

Category	Positive Statements	Negative Statements
Discussion points by partner	Dissuaded me from quitting	Expressed concerns that treatment successes may only be temporary
	Motivated me to keep going	Complained about me leaving the bedroom during the night
	Made positive comments about my improved mood	Insisted bedtime routines should stay the same
	Asked about the content of sessions	Said I was really hard to live with because I was so tired
	Encouraged me to attend sessions	Voiced concerns that I was not getting better
	Asked me to teach them my distraction techniques	Said I should stay in bed and try to sleep
	Mentioned that I am nicer since starting CBT-I	Refused to remove visible clock/alarm clock
	Did not complain about new sleep routines even though they were disruptive	Complained about changes to the bedroom
	Told me I look better/healthier	Encouraged me to go to bed if I was falling asleep
	Reminded me to complete my sleep diary	Made unhelpful comments about having even less energy (physical)
	Made positive comments about my improved energy	Told me off if I deviated from your instructions
	Asked what they could do to help me	Complained about the new routines
	Reminded me to stop working before bedtime	Encouraged me to spend more time in bed at the weekend
	Made positive comments about our improved relationship	Made negative comments about me having even less energy (mental)
	Reminded me to complete my cognitive diary	Wanted to see everything I was doing including my diaries
		Said my distraction techniques were strange
Actions by partner	Woke me if I was having a nap/dozing	Allowed me to sleep in occasionally
	Stopped using technology in the bedroom	Will not see someone about their snoring
	Helped me find things to do at night	Would not keep me company at night
	Stayed up later with me at night	Used computer/tablet/phone in bedroom
	Gave me rewards to keep me going	Wanted to talk about sleep and my insomnia just before bed
	Provided physical help with making changes	Would close the windows overnight
	Got up at the same time as me in the morning	Interrupted me during my distraction techniques
	Gave me space to do my homework	
	Changed their presleep routine to fit in with mine	
	Did our relaxation exercises together	
	Made me lots of noncaffeinated drinks	
	Purchased me magazines/books to read in my wind down time	
	Purchased me fruit teas	

(continued on next page)

Table 1
(continued)

Category	Positive Statements	Negative Statements
Beliefs of partner	Believed in my ability to cope with CBT-I	Does not believe in CBT-I/talking therapies
	Understands why sleep hygiene is important	Thinks insomnia is not a proper illness
	Provided emotional support throughout the therapy	Failed to understand my treatment
	Understands the reason for sleep restriction	Thought that I should quit
	Would know what to do to help me prevent a relapse	
	Understands why sleep is so important to me	

factor on the other. This may help determine whether, as is the case with some other conditions, CBT-I should be prioritized over addressing any relationship concerns or issues. Alternatively, whether a hybrid form of relationship-based therapy, which considers sleep—potentially adding elements of CBT-I—is warranted.

With respect to outcomes, a final consideration here is to ask the question, what is meaningful in terms of the treatment of insomnia in this context? Although some outcome measures, such as those associated with feasibility (uptake, attrition, completion), are important to understand the acceptability and tolerability of the intervention itself, traditional treatment outcome measures focus on changes in symptoms and insomnia status (eg, sleep diary data, psychometrics—such as the Insomnia Severity Index or Pittsburgh Sleep Quality Index). This latter category, however, may be quite sensitive but lack specificity. For example, where aggregated values/scores along a broad spectrum of outcomes are usually derived; is a change in daytime functioning more or less valuable to the patient than a change in the number of nocturnal awakenings. In the context of the present discussion, one area that has received no attention, to date, but may be fruitful, is changes in family functioning, satisfaction or relationship dynamics as a result of CBT-I. To what extent are these factors important/meaningful to the patient?

SUMMARY

Sleep and relationship functioning are interesting bedfellows with one affecting the other and vice versa. Moreover, these relationships are accentuated in the face of both poorer sleep and/or poorer relationship functioning. That said, the research in the area of insomnia and relationship status and functioning is limited. Even more so is the influence partners may have in the context of CBT-I. Although it seems that a role could exist for partner inclusion as an adjuvant to CBT-I, there is still a great deal of research needed beforehand.

CLINICS CARE POINTS

- When assessing an individual for insomnia disorder, you should ask about the influence of partners.
- If partners are likely to be influential to CBT-I, invite them to the first clinical session.
- If partners seem to be a barrier to treatment adherence, during CBT-I, consider a joint session with them and the patient.

ACKNOWLEDGMENTS

None.

DISCLOSURE

The authors have nothing to disclose.

REFERENCES

1. Qaseem A, Kansagara D, Forciea MA, et al. Management of chronic insomnia disorder in adults: a clinical practice guideline from the American College of Physicians. Ann Intern Med 2016;165(2): 125–33.
2. Riemann D, Baglioni C, Bassetti C, et al. European guideline for the diagnosis and treatment of insomnia. J Sleep Res 2017;26(6):675–700.
3. Natsky AN, Vakulin A, Chai-Coetzer CL, et al. Economic evaluation of cognitive behavioural therapy

for insomnia (CBT-I) for improving health outcomes in adult populations: a systematic review. Sleep Med Rev 2020;54:101351.

4. Schutte-Rodin S, Broch L, Buysse D, et al. Clinical guideline for the evaluation and management of chronic insomnia in adults. J Clin Sleep Med 2008; 4(5):487–504.

5. Morin CM, Hauri PJ, Espie CA, et al. Nonpharmacologic treatment of chronic insomnia. Sleep 1999; 22(8):1134–56.

6. Morin CM, Bootzin RR, Buysse DJ, et al. Psychological and behavioral treatment of insomnia: update of the recent evidence (1998–2004). Sleep 2006; 29(11):1398–414.

7. Pillai V, Roth T, Drake CL. Towards quantitative cutoffs for insomnia: how current diagnostic criteria mischaracterize remission. Sleep Med 2016;26:62–8.

8. van Straten A, Lancee J. Digital cognitive behavioural therapy for insomnia: the answer to a major public health issue? Lancet Digital Health 2020;2(8): e381–2.

9. Ong JC, Kuo TF, Manber R. Who is at risk for dropout from group cognitive-behavior therapy for insomnia? J psychosomatic Res 2008;64(4):419–25.

10. Koffel E, Amundson E, Polusny G, et al. You're missing out on something great": patient and provider perspectives on increasing the use of cognitive behavioral therapy for insomnia. Behav Sleep Med 2020;18(3):358–71.

11. Gardiner A, Stanley N. 0527 the uptake of a free digital CBTi programme in a large commercial organisation. Sleep 2020;43:A201–2.

12. Matthews EE, Arnedt JT, McCarthy MS, et al. Adherence to cognitive behavioral therapy for insomnia: a systematic review. Sleep Med Rev 2013;17(6): 453–64.

13. Grandner MA, Hale L, Moore M, et al. Mortality associated with short sleep duration: the evidence, the possible mechanisms, and the future. Sleep Med Rev 2010;14(3):191–203.

14. Meadows R. The 'negotiated night': an embodied conceptual framework for the sociological study of sleep. Sociological Rev 2005;53(2):240–54.

15. Meadows R, Arber S, Venn S, et al. Exploring the interdependence of couples' rest-wake cycles: an actigraphic study. Chronobiology Int 2009;26(1):80–92.

16. Pankhurst FP, Home JA. The influence of bed partners on movement during sleep. Sleep 1994;17(4): 308–15.

17. Luyster FS. Impact of obstructive sleep apnea and its treatments on partners: a literature review. J Clin Sleep Med 2017;13(3):467–77.

18. Ye L, Malhotra A, Kayser K, et al. Spousal involvement and CPAP adherence: a dyadic perspective. Sleep Med Rev 2015;19:67–74.

19. Rogojanski J, Carney CE, Monson CM. Interpersonal factors in insomnia: a model for integrating bed partners into cognitive behavioral therapy for insomnia. Sleep Med Rev 2013;17(1):55–64.

20. Troxel WM, Robles TF, Hall M, et al. Marital quality and the marital bed: examining the covariation between relationship quality and sleep. Sleep Med Rev 2007;11(5):389–404.

21. Lalley-Chareczko L, Segal A, Perlis ML, et al. Sleep disturbance partially mediates the relationship between intimate partner violence and physical/mental health in women and men. J interpersonal violence 2017;32(16):2471–95.

22. Siltala HP, Holma JM, Hallman M. Family violence and mental health in a sample of Finnish health care professionals: the mediating role of perceived sleep quality. Scand J caring Sci 2019;33(1): 231–43.

23. Kotronoulas G, Wengström Y, Kearney N. Sleep and sleep-wake disturbances in care recipient-caregiver dyads in the context of a chronic illness: a critical review of the literature. J Pain Symptom Manage 2013; 45(3):579–94.

24. Brewster GS, Bliwise D, Epps F, et al. Dyadic factors that associate with insomnia in caregivers of persons living with dementia. Innovation in Aging 2019;3(Suppl 1):S367.

25. Shaffer KM, Garland SN, Mao JJ, et al. Insomnia among cancer caregivers: a proposal for tailored cognitive behavioral therapy. J psychotherapy integration 2018;28(3):275.

26. Strawbridge WJ, Shema SJ, Roberts RE. Impact of spouses' sleep problems on partners. Sleep 2004; 27(3):527–31.

27. Zee PC, Sheehan D, Steinberg K, et al. Insomnia Impacts the patient and the household: perceptions of the burden of insomnia on next-day functioning. Sleep Med 2019;64:S129–30.

28. Revenson TA, Marín-Chollom AM, Rundle AG, et al. Hey Mr. Sandman: dyadic effects of anxiety, depressive symptoms and sleep among married couples. J Behav Med 2016;39(2):225–32.

29. Carney CE, Ulmer C, Edinger JD, et al. Assessing depression symptoms in those with insomnia: an examination of the beck depression inventory second edition (BDI-II). J Psychiatr Res 2009;43(5):576–82.

30. Shih YC, Han SH, Burr JA. Are spouses' sleep problems a mechanism through which health is compromised? Evidence regarding insomnia and heart disease. Ann Behav Med 2019;53(4):345–57.

31. Walters EM, Phillips AJ, Boardman JM, et al. Vulnerability and resistance to sleep disruption by a partner: a study of bed-sharing couples. Sleep Health 2020;6(4):506–12.

32. Gunn HE, Buysse DJ, Hasler BP, et al. Sleep concordance in couples is associated with relationship characteristics. Sleep 2015;38(6):933–9.

33. Troxel WM, Braithwaite SR, Sandberg JG, et al. Does improving marital quality improve sleep?

Results from a marital therapy trial. Behav Sleep Med 2017;15(4):330–43.

34. Sedov I, Madsen JW, Goodman SH, et al. Couples' treatment preferences for insomnia experienced during pregnancy. Families, Syst Health 2019; 37(1):46.

35. Araújo T, Lemyre A, Vallières A, et al. Sociocultural variations of coping strategies for sleep difficulties in couple relationships in Canada and Brazil. Sleep and Hypnosis 2019;21(2):158–69.

36. Kamen C, Garland SN, Heckler CE, et al. Social support, insomnia, and adherence to cognitive behavioral therapy for insomnia after cancer treatment. Behav Sleep Med 2019;17(1):70–80.

37. Dyrberg H, Juel A, Kragh M. Experience of treatment and adherence to cognitive behavioral therapy for insomnia for patients with depression: an interview study. Behav Sleep Med 2021;19(4):481–91.

38. Lange A, Waterman DÉ, Kerkhof G. Sleep-wake patterns of partners. Perceptual Mot skills 1998;86(3_suppl):1141–2.

39. Larson JH, Crane DR, Smith CW. Morning and night couples: the effect of wake and sleep patterns on marital adjustment. J Marital Fam Ther 1991;17(1):53–65.

40. Adams BN, Cromwell RE. Morning and night people in the family: a preliminary statement. Fam Coordinator 1978;27(1):5–13.

41. Ellis JG. The one week insomnia cure. London: Vermillion Press; 2017.

42. Ellis JG, Deary V, Troxel WM. The role of perceived partner alliance on efficacy of CBT-I: preliminary findings from the Partner Alliance in Insomnia Research Study (PAIRS). Behav Sleep Med 2015; 13(1):64–72.

43. Gold MA, Dahl RE. Using Motivational Interviewing to facilitate healthier sleep-related behaviors in adolescents. In: Perlis ML, Aloia M, Kuhn B, editors. Behavioral treatments for sleep disorders: a comprehensive primer of behavioral sleep medicine interventions. Waltham, MA: Academic Press; 2010. p. 367–82.

44. Mellor A, Hamill K, Jenkins MM, et al. Partner-assisted cognitive behavioural therapy for insomnia versus cognitive behavioural therapy for insomnia: a randomised controlled trial. Trials 2019;20(1):1–12.

Paradoxic Intention as an Adjunct Treatment to Cognitive Behavioral Therapy for Insomnia

Markus Jansson-Fröjmark, PhD[a],*, Christina Sandlund, PhD[b],
Annika Norell-Clarke, PhD[c,d,e]

KEYWORDS

- Insomnia • Cognitive behavior therapy • Paradoxic intention • Performance anxiety
- Sleep intention

KEY POINTS

- PI is an evidence-based single-component treatment of insomnia that has the potential to reduce sleep onset latency and the number of awakenings, by instructing patients to stay awake for as long as possible in their beds.
- The original theory is that PI reduces sleep-related performance anxiety, which allows for natural sleep initiation processes to take place, but there are other potential mechanisms, which the article also describes.
- Owing to the lack of studies regarding for whom PI works, clinicians' use of PI in the treatment of insomnia should be based on theoretic knowledge, clinical experience and the patient's needs, resources, and preferences, as well as available treatment options.
- If PI is given as a part of CBT-I, the clinician must consider the potential theoretic or practical clashes with other treatment components, such as stimulus control and sleep restriction.
- Future studies are needed to cover the knowledge gap on the effects of PI in populations in which CBT-I may be unsuitable, the effects of PI on daytime symptoms, how long the effects last for, patients' adherence, side effects, and mechanisms of change.

BACKGROUND

One of the first psychological treatment components for insomnia disorder that was described in the literature is paradoxic intention (PI). As early as the 1970s, Ascher and Efran[1] reported on this new treatment technique and the efficacy of PI in 5 cases with sleep-onset insomnia.[1] The investigators described that they instructed 5 participants with insomnia to "try to remain awake," rather than to focus on trying to fall asleep. In the first case series, PI was used for 2 weeks, resulting in a marked reduction in sleep onset latency. Another interesting finding to emerge from the case reports was that the patients reported difficulty in adhering to PI because they had fallen asleep too quickly: a paradoxic effect.

Although the basic instruction of staying awake has remained unchanged, the rationale for PI has varied over the years (**Table 1**). In the first

[a] Department of Clinical Neuroscience, Centre for Psychiatry Research, Karolinska Institutet & Stockholm Health Care Services, Competence Center for Psychotherapy Research and Education, Liljeholmstorget 7, Stockholm 117 63, Sweden; [b] Department of Neurobiology, Care Sciences and Society, Academic Primary Health Care Centre, Karolinska Institutet, Solnavägen 1 E, Stockholm 113 65, Sweden; [c] Centre for Research on Children's and Adolescent's Mental Health, Karlstad University, 651 88 Karlstad, Sweden; [d] Department of Law, Psychology and Social Work, Örebro University, Box 1252, Örebro 701 12, Sweden; [e] Faculty of Health Sciences, Kristianstad University, Kristianstad SE–291 88, Sweden
* Corresponding author.
E-mail address: markus.jansson-frojmark@ki.se

Sleep Med Clin 18 (2023) 9–19
https://doi.org/10.1016/j.jsmc.2022.10.001

Table 1
Description of different versions of paradoxic intention

Name	Core Instructions (Brief Summaries)	Comment
Paradoxic intention: type A instructions	Lie comfortably in bed, in a dark room, with your eyes open. Try to remain awake for as long as possible, without engaging in sleep-incompatible activities	This is the original version, which is considered "core" PI[2]
Paradoxic intention with reframing instructions: type B instructions	Lie comfortably in bed, in a dark room, with your eyes open. Try to remain awake for as long as possible, without engaging in sleep-incompatible activities. Observe your thoughts, so that they can be used in future psychotherapy sessions to improve your insomnia treatment	This version has mainly been used as an active control condition in PI studies or other insomnia treatment studies[4,5,7]
Paradoxic intention combined with relaxation instructions	Lie comfortably in bed, in a dark room, with your eyes open. Use relaxation exercises for longer than you would usually, even if it means fighting off the urge to sleep. A more relaxed state will allow you to fall asleep better	To the best of our knowledge, this version of PI has only been tested as an addition to established relaxation exercises, which had been previously unsuccessful in shortening the patients' sleep onset[1]
Paradoxic intention with "give up trying" instructions	Lie comfortably in bed, in a dark room, with your eyes open. Give up trying to fall asleep, without engaging in sleep-incompatible activities. This will make your time in bed less distressed, and you will be more rested in the morning	Only found in 1 study.[6] It is remarkably similar to later ACT approaches to sleeplessness.

Abbreviation: ACT, acceptance and commitment therapy.

empirical study by Ascher and Efran,[1] the core instruction of PI was "try to remain awake," and the rationale given to 3 of the patients was that observing thoughts before sleep onset might provide information on how to deliver therapy more effectively. Another type of rationale, which was delivered to the remaining 2 patients in the study by Ascher and Efran,[1] was to instruct patients to resist the urge to sleep and to apply relaxation in bed to reach a satisfactory level of relaxation and subsequently to be able to fall asleep. A third type of PI was also described in an article by Ascher and Turner,[2] in which patients were instructed to apply PI while keeping their eyes open and lying comfortably in bed or in a dark room (also known as Type A instructions). Based on how PI is used in later studies, we draw the conclusion that the last rationale by Ascher and Turner[2] seems to be the one that nowadays is

regarded as "true" PI, for example, described by Espie[3]; this also means that the first 2 types, which involve observing thoughts or applying relaxation, seem outdated in the treatment literature.

How is PI practiced today? Although the use of PI is likely to differ across clinicians and settings, we propose that the approach by Espie[3] is comprehensive yet simple. Espie[3] suggests that the first step with the patient is to elaborate on a good sleeper's routines, mainly that the normal sleeper does not deliberately or anxiously try to influence sleep. It is also recommended in the approach to ask the patient to complete a sleep effort scale (eg, the Glasgow Sleep Effort Scale), but fill out the 7 items pretending to be a good sleeper, so that the patient sees low or nonexistent sleep effort in practice. The next step is to consider the patient's insomnia as a "sleep effort syndrome," a state in which the patient sees sleep as an effort and is preoccupied with falling asleep. Espie[3] proposes that drawing parallels to other problems or situations might be helpful at this stage, for example, by contrasting sleeping at home and somewhere else, trying too hard when performing a sport, or attempting to remove a thought or tune from one's head. The next and final step is when PI is introduced and implemented. In this step, Espie[3] mentions 2 methods for giving up trying to sleep. Method 1 consists of a "giving up trying" approach, labeled "turning the tables." In this method, acceptance and mindfulness are central ingredients, for example, accepting insomnia as a part of life and viewing wakefulness as an opportunity. Method 1 takes inspiration from the "give up trying" approach that was developed by Fogle and Dyal[6] (see **Table 1**). Method 2 is more clearly paradoxic, in which the patient encourages unwanted insomnia symptoms by trying to stay awake. Method 2 also advises the patient to lie comfortably in bed with eyes open, give up sleep effort and concern about being awake, and continuously repeating the core instruction of trying to stay awake. Both methods are thus "giving up trying" approaches at the core, however, with different means to get there. In method 2, the patient should go to bed at a normal time when feeling sleepy and turn the lights off, followed by trying to stay awake.

Just as the methods of PI have varied over time, the theoretic foundations of PI have also developed. In the beginning, PI was centered on the idea that patients with insomnia are unable to grasp that sleep is an involuntary physiologic process, and that they, therefore, muster their full effort to initiate sleep.[1] Furthermore, Ascher and Efran[1] suggested that the intentional effort to try to fall asleep leads to frustration and activation of the autonomic nervous system, which interferes with sleep initiation. As a result, a vicious cycle has been formed, in which self-monitoring, heightened arousal, performance anxiety, sleep effort, and failure to fall asleep impact upon one another. In this original proposal, PI is assumed to work by reducing performance anxiety.[1] In a subsequent model, PI was viewed in the light of the attention-intention-effort (AIE) model.[8] In the AIE conceptualization, it is proposed that selective attention to threatening sleep cues, such as a beating heart and external noise, triggers explicit intention to sleep, which leads to the inhibition of normal dearousal.[9] As a result, the amplified intention to sleep triggers direct and indirect sleep effort, such as actively trying to sleep and extending time in bed. In the AIE model, PI is seen as an intervention that manipulates the intensified sleep intention by remaining passively awake or by

giving up any direct intention to try to fall asleep. Besides performance anxiety and sleep intention as theoretic foundations for PI, there are a few additional suggested mechanisms. First, PI could also be viewed as enabling exposure to learned feared stimuli in bed[10]. Lundh[10] suggests that certain "awake" stimuli, such as the alarm clock next to bed or the trapped air in the bedroom, may trigger activation of the central nervous system, for example, by increasing heart rate and thereby prolonging sleep initiation. By being instructed to stay awake in bed, the effects from the conditioned stimuli might habituate, as the patient perceives them fully without attempting to "avoid" or "flee" (as by trying to fall asleep). A second additional mechanism, not yet described in the literature to our knowledge, is sleep drive. We suggest that PI may work, at least partly, through the buildup of sleep pressure when patients with insomnia experience frequent and extended awakenings at night, that is, objective sleep loss. As a result, we propose that sleep pressure is an important establishing condition or mechanism through which PI influences insomnia symptoms, in particular sleep initiation difficulties. Third, acceptance of unwanted, inner experiences, such as distressing thoughts, negative feelings, and aversive bodily sensations, may also be a mechanism through which PI works.[11] In the context of PI, it is possible that the instruction of "try to remain awake" enables patients with insomnia to adopt a stance where the struggle to fall asleep is abandoned, and instead means rehearsing acceptance of unpleasant, inner experiences.

PI shares some features with other therapy techniques, which should be distinguished from PI. For example, cognitive therapy for insomnia can include the "fear of bad sleep" behavioral experiment in which patients test their beliefs about what will happen if they get less sleep than they think they need[12]; this commonly means planning an evening in which the patient goes to bed later than usual, gets up at their usual time, and evaluates the consequences the day after. The difference between PI and this behavioral experiment is that in the former patients are instructed to be (passively) awake in bed, whereas in the latter patients are active in one way or another outside their bedrooms. Also, the behavioral experiment is usually introduced late in the treatment, when patients have developed skills to handle insomnia and had some success in improving their sleep,[12] whereas PI is introduced as the only technique or introduced early in CBT-I.

Another therapy technique that is similar to PI is the use of *acceptance* in bed while waiting for sleep to come. This technique stems from Acceptance and Commitment Therapy (ACT) paradigms, which have started to gain recognition as an insomnia treatment.[13] Instead of trying to fall asleep, patients are instructed to manage presleep distress by ceasing the struggle for control over sleep or thoughts, and instead practice acceptance of whatever thoughts, feelings, and sensations may arise. Falling asleep quickly is not the goal, although it might be a side effect. This approach is similar to one of the types of PI administration (also known as Type B), in which patients are instructed to focus on their thoughts and gather information for the therapist on their pre-sleep thought content,[1] which might make a person more of an objective observer than a fully immersed "thinker" and in turn work through the same mechanisms as acceptance. It should be noted that the acceptance technique does not include instructions to report back to the therapist. In some studies, the Type B version includes the creation of exposure hierarchies of distressing thoughts and desensitization training during the following sessions, although we have not been able to find support for this use outside of clinical studies where Type B was the control condition. It should be mentioned that one early PI study used a "give up trying" instructions (see also **Table 1**), which seem analogous to later acceptance techniques, because the goal was "a genuine acceptance of the status quo." Patients were informed that by giving up efforts to fall asleep, they would be less anxious and feel more comfortable about being awake during the night; they were explicitly informed not to expect this approach to affect their sleep.[6]

Research

The evidence base of PI has been assessed several times over the years. The American Academy of Sleep Medicine (AASM) has conducted 3 reviews since the 1990s. The first AASM review identified 6 studies that had examined the efficacy of PI for patients with sleep-onset insomnia.[14] Although 4 studies in the review from 1999 demonstrated that PI was more efficacious than control conditions in reducing sleep onset latency, 2 trials did not observe significant differences between PI and control groups. Using other passive and active control conditions as comparisons, meta-analytic calculations demonstrated that the between-group effect sizes were d = 0.46 for total sleep time as an outcome, d = 0.63 for sleep onset latency, d = 0.73 for number of awakenings, and d = 0.81 for wake after sleep onset. As a whole, the AASM review from 1999 stated that PI is an

empirically supported intervention. An updated review from the AASM[15] also categorized PI as a well-established treatment. Several methodological and statistical limitations hamper the conclusions from the AASM reviews,[14,15] such as including only examining trials up until 2004, only using 2 databases when identifying relevant studies, only examining the efficacy of PI based on nighttime symptoms, unclear reporting of methodological and statistical aspects in the quantitative assessment of PI, and using outdated criteria for classifying treatments as well-established treatments and probably efficacious treatments. The latest AASM report[16] consists of a systematic review approach combined with meta-analytic estimations and a summary assessment of the evidence of various behavioral and psychological treatments for insomnia disorder. The review aimed to determine clinically significant improvements based on outcomes the investigators considered critical and important. Only 2 of 5 reviewed studies on PI met the criteria and were included in the meta-analysis. The report investigators conclude that the overall quality of evidence is very low for the use of PI due to imprecision, inconsistency, and risk of bias,[16] and they did not recommend PI as a single-component treatment in their succeeding clinical practice guideline for behavioral and psychological treatments for insomnia.[17]

Two of this article's authors performed a narrative review in 2018, which concluded that PI has empirical support for insomnia.[18] Because the narrative review did not evaluate the efficacy of PI in quantitative terms and did not explicitly discriminate between outcomes (eg, nighttime and daytime symptoms), we, together with colleagues, performed a systematic review and meta-analysis of the efficacy of PI.[19] Based on 10 included trials, the meta-analytic calculations showed that PI resulted in large improvements in central insomnia symptoms, relative to passive comparators. More specifically, PI was largely superior to passive comparators in reducing sleep initiation and the number of awakenings (Hedge's g = 0.82–1.71). Compared with active comparators, the improvements were less pronounced, but still moderate for some key outcomes, for example, on difficulty falling asleep (g = 0.69) and number of awakenings (g = 0.55). PI also resulted in large decreases in sleep-related performance anxiety (g = 1.04), one of several proposed mechanisms of change for PI. A limitation this last review shares with its predecessors is that the only evaluated measure of sleep-maintenance insomnia is the number of awakenings. Although fewer awakenings might be analogous to lessened sleep maintenance issues, the duration of un-wanted time awake is unknown and might be thus unchanged or even increased after treatment. This fallacy in the reviews is due to how sleep maintenance was measured in the included studies. As a result, conclusions regarding the effects from PI on sleep-maintenance insomnia are limited to the number of awakenings.

Although the latest AASM review and meta-analysis reports the quality of evidence for PI as very low, there are, as mentioned earlier, other reviews and meta-analyses that demonstrate the efficacy of PI to be of clinical value. Besides the potential clinical benefits of PI, there might, however, also be negative effects following administration of PI. To our knowledge, there is only 1 trial that has specifically assessed and reported on adverse events or deterioration. More specifically, a case series with 6 patients with sleep-onset insomnia[20] reported that sleep onset increased for 3 of 6 patients using PI. The investigators speculate that the deterioration observed in the 3 patients might be due to PI in itself, that PI might be less appropriate for those with severe sleep-onset insomnia, and that it was "too easy" for the 3 patients to remain awake using PI. However, a common denominator for many therapies is that positive outcomes partly depend on the participants' ability to endure discomfort in the beginning of therapy. For example, in sleep restriction therapy, participants must withstand increased sleep performance anxiety and sleepiness before experiences of improved sleep and daytime functioning.[21] Moreover, exposure to fears is a common intervention for anxiety disorders,[22] and parallels can be drawn to PI and fears of not falling asleep. However, because none of the remaining PI studies systematically assessed adverse events or deterioration, more research is warranted to examine whether PI produces negative effects among patients with insomnia in general or in subgroups of patients.

As a whole, we argue that PI should be viewed as a potentially efficacious intervention in the context of insomnia. Before more firm conclusions can be made, more rigorous trials are needed that include patients with a current definition of insomnia disorder, use a broad assessment of clinical benefit and potential negative effects, and explore moderators and theory-based mechanisms of change.

Clinical Relevance

The relevance of implementing PI in clinical settings could be argued to stem from 2 sources: one based on the strengths of PI and one based on the limitations of CBT-I. The clinical benefits of PI have already been reported on earlier, with the most marked outcomes improved being reductions in sleep initiation and maintenance problems. In fact, if the efficacy of PI is compared, as demonstrated in the meta-analysis performed by Jansson-Fröjmark,[19] with other cognitive and behavioral interventions (eg, CBT-I, relaxation, stimulus control, psychoeducation, and sleep restriction) for insomnia disorder, as shown in a recent meta-analysis,[23] there are clear clinical benefits of PI. Relative to other cognitive and behavioral interventions, PI results in larger effect sizes (relative to passive comparators) on sleep onset latency (0.57 vs 0.82), number of awakenings (0.28 vs 1.10), and total sleep time (0.16 vs 0.51), but a smaller effect size on sleep efficiency (0.71 vs 0.00). Although comparisons of this sort are difficult, a tentative conclusion might be that PI has at least similar effects as other evidence-based, psychological interventions on sleep/insomnia.

The recent review and meta-analysis[19] also demonstrated that PI results in a large reduction in sleep-related performance anxiety, relative to passive comparators; this is a finding that could be suggestive of the fact that reduced performance anxiety is a mechanism of change for PI and possibly also an etiologic factor, which is an expected result according to theory.[1] If sleep-related performance anxiety is indeed a maintaining factor for insomnia disorder in general, this could strengthen the clinical relevance of PI. More specifically, patients with elevated sleep-related performance anxiety could be offered PI as a first-line or at least an early intervention during CBT-I. If this proposed pathway is to be implemented in clinical settings, a rigorous randomized controlled trial is first warranted. Another advantage of PI is that it may be relatively easy for clinicians with little or no psychotherapy training (eg, physicians, nurses, and physiotherapists) to learn to deliver, and to use in a variety of clinical settings, such as primary health care, nursing homes, and psychiatric settings.

Another way to underscore the clinical relevance of PI is to focus on the limitations of CBT-I. Despite the effectiveness of CBT-I, the AASM reviews from 1999[14] and 2021[16] both concluded that about a half will fail to achieve clinically meaningful improvements.[16] Adjunct interventions for insomnia are thus in place and may help meet individual treatment needs.

Although access to CBT-I has increased in recent years, its long, multicomponent nature makes it challenging to implement and resource demanding in clinical settings. Digital solutions can help increase access to CBT-I,[24] but they do not suit everyone.[25] Moreover, no matter whether it is delivered in person or digitally, CBT-I requires active engagement in methods that can be mentally and physically challenging, and not everyone is able or motivated to engage fully in treatment.[26] Some CBT-I components, such as the core components sleep restriction and stimulus control, might also be less appropriate for certain patients or subgroups. Initially, sleep restriction therapy increases daytime sleepiness and impairs vigilance[27]; this may make CBT-I inappropriate for certain groups of people, such as heavy machinery operators, professional drivers, people predisposed to mania/hypomania, and people with seizure disorders.[17] Moreover, sleep restriction requires prerequisites for regular sleep habits, and is therefore not suitable for shift workers. Stimulus control therapy may increase the risk of falls in certain populations, such as older adults with frailty and people who use hypnotics.[17] PI may thus be useful as a second-line treatment of people for whom CBT-I is not appropriate or suitable.

Considerations

In this section, some considerations regarding the use of PI are suggested. The first consideration pertains to for whom PI could be used and for how long. The later considerations regard the use of PI as a single adjunctive therapy or as a component of CBT-I.

Paradoxic intention: for whom and for how long?

Owing to the complete lack of research teasing out how to match patients to treatments in this area, we would argue for a more theory-driven approach when considering PI as a potential adjunct treatment. Based on the potential mechanisms of change for PI, as mentioned in the background, there are at least 5 factors/models that could be of relevance; performance anxiety, sleep intention, exposure, sleep drive, and acceptance. First and second, for patients with elevated sleep-related performance anxiety or sleep intention, PI could be an effective adjunct or second-line intervention. The obvious candidate would be a patient with sleep-onset insomnia who acts as if sleep initiation should and can be actively controlled. In a similar vein, PI could function as a test of patients' dysfunctional beliefs about their ability to cope with sleeplessness: similar to the "fear of poor sleep" as described by Ree and Harvey.[12] Third, PI could also work through exposure to learned, feared stimuli in the bed or bedroom,[10] that is, "awake" properties. As mentioned previously, it

is not uncommon that patients report that objects or qualities in the bedroom are able to trigger activation of the central nervous system, for example, by increasing heart rate and thereby prolonging sleep initiation. Fourth, we also suggest that sleep drive is a necessary ingredient in the efficacy of PI. For example, a patient who has built up an extensive sleep drive during the past days (eg, through frequent and extended awakenings at night) is, according to us, a good candidate for PI, whereas a patient with limited sleep drive (eg, through a couple of good nights of sleep) is a less optimal candidate for PI. Fifth, patients struggling with falling asleep and not allowing unwanted, inner experiences, such as intrusive thoughts, to be part of the daily experience may also be good candidates for PI. For such a candidate, the PI instruction of "try to remain awake" might result in less of a struggle with sleep and more of accepting the present, "awake" moment.

Moreover, it is possible that persons with sleep-onset insomnia, as opposed to sleep-maintenance insomnia, will have a more positive response from PI, because sleep drive is generally stronger during sleep onset and is reduced during nightly awakenings because of a couple of hours sleep. In the recent review and meta-analysis on PI,[19] 7 studies included participants with sleep-onset insomnia, and 3 studies included participants with mixed sleep-onset and sleep-maintenance insomnia. Further research is needed to determine if PI is more effective in sleep-onset insomnia than in sleep-maintenance insomnia. Also, future studies should report outcomes on both the number of awakenings and the total time awake after first sleep onset. In the context of sleep drive, it should also be underscored that other treatment components, such as sleep restriction, are viable routes when patients present with a significant sleep drive. The use of PI might also have the benefit of preventing patients from using sleep-disturbing behaviors in bed and exposing them to their own thoughts, feelings, and bodily sensations. For patients who always "need" to be occupied by something, and use devices (eg, smartphones) to fill their unwanted sleepless time, PI might give them a chance to experience what lying in bed without distractions might be like.

The length of time that PI should be administered to demonstrate an effect is another clinical consideration. In most studies, PI is instructed at the first session, and the following 2 to 3 sessions are devoted to problem solving and fine tuning. In a few studies, patients were cautioned not to expect improved sleep until after a few weeks of treatment.[2,5] This caveat might be wise because one study reported that a third of the participants experienced longer sleep onset latencies during the first week of PI, although sleep onset had shortened by the end of treatment.[28] This report corresponds with our clinical experience, wherein some report prolonged sleep onset after PI. (Regrettably, we do not know how their trajectories would have played out because our patients were instructed to try another technique instead, during comprehensive CBT-I with new techniques being introduced most weeks).

Paradoxic intention as an adjunctive treatment to cognitive behavioral therapy for insomnia

Given the current evidence base, it is reasonable to view CBT-I as a first-line intervention for insomnia disorder, and PI as second option after CBT-I has been considered or attempted, just like pharmacotherapy in the European guidelines for insomnia treatment.[29]

The questions then are under what circumstances PI could be seen as an adjunct treatment to CBT-I and how PI could be implemented. It is important to emphasize that PI is not commonly considered as an ingredient in current CBT-I,[19] although some studies have included it.[30,31] Instead, standard CBT-I is commonly described as comprising psychoeducation, sleep restriction, stimulus control, sleep hygiene instructions, dearousal components, and cognitive components.[29] At present, there is little research support for PI to be used before or concurrently with CBT-I. Rather, PI may be used for patients who do not respond at all or inadequately to standard CBT-I, because it initially was tested on patients who did not respond to behavioral therapies for insomnia.[1] Decisions to implement PI for patients who do not respond successfully to standard CBT-I should be based on a thorough screening for maintaining factors of insomnia that confirms the presence of sleep performance anxiety or sleep effort, for example, by using the 7-item Glasgow Sleep Effort Scale[8] or other potential sleep-disturbing mechanisms that PI has the potential to affect. A new treatment rationale based on the assessment and the patients' preferences could then be tailored, which may include PI if relevant.

Paradoxic intention as a part of cognitive behavioral therapy for insomnia

Although uncommon in the literature, PI has been included in some effective CBT-I therapies.[30,31] When using PI as a component of CBT-I, one needs to consider that some CBT-I components might be difficult to integrate with PI, because the rationales are incompatible. We argue that this difficulty is specifically salient for 3 treatment components: sleep restriction, stimulus control, and dearousal components. First, the core of sleep restriction—restriction of time in bed—is not easily assimilated with PI.[32] In fact, "restricting time in bed" means less hours in bed and thereby limited opportunities for PI to take place. Second, the first 3 instructions in stimulus control are not in line with PI, namely, "Lie down to go to sleep only when you are sleepy," "Do not use your bed for anything except sleep," and "If you find yourself unable to fall asleep, get up and go into another room." The mismatch in key treatment elements between PI and sleep restriction and stimulus control are so large, leading us to think that they are not compatible to implement at the same time. Instead, we advise clinicians to use these 2 treatment components in a sequential manner, for example, first implementing sleep restriction and then PI, or vice versa, as in the studies that have included PI in CBT.[30,31]

Dearousal components, such as relaxation training and mindfulness, might be more easily integrated with PI as long as they are practiced and implemented outside bed. However, if the therapeutic aim is that the patient uses these components in bed, a mismatch is possible, although it should be noted that PI has been successfully added to relaxation.[1] Cognitive techniques may be easier than behavioral techniques to combine with PI. For instance, if using the reframing version of PI (instructions to stay awake to observe one's thoughts) this could have the added benefit of gathering information on the patient's dysfunctional beliefs about sleep, negative repetitive thinking, and other sleep-disturbing thought content or inner behaviors.

To date, studies have not investigated whether including PI in CBT-I improves treatment results. However, a qualitative study,[26] exploring experiences of group CBT-I in primary health care,[31] has found that participants may experience benefits when PI is included as a component of CBT-I. In that study,[31] PI was introduced as a 1-night behavioral experiment before the introduction of stimulus control and sleep restriction. The findings indicated that participants increased their ability to dedramatize sleep and sleeplessness by accepting the situation and letting go of the idea that they had to force themselves to sleep.[26] Thus, PI may have served as a learning experience, at least for some participants. However, participants did not name PI as an important treatment component. One even stated that PI was not useful at all, because she fell asleep immediately, and thus felt she failed to follow the instructions (ie, try to stay awake in bed). Albeit an amusing anecdote, this patient's experience may be related to

Table 2
Components in cognitive behavioral therapy for insomnia that primary health care patients reported as useful directly after therapy and 1 year after therapy

Components	Posttreatment (n = 96) % (n)	12 mo Posttreatment (n = 69) % (n)
Psychoeducation	85.4 (76)	71.0 (49)
Sleep hygiene	39.6 (38)	66.7 (46)
Breathing exercise	62.5 (60)	42.0 (29)
Paradoxic intention	30.2 (29)	23.2 (16)
Worry time	29.2 (28)	7.2 (5)
Stimulus control	17.7 (17)	30.4 (21)
Sleep restriction	71.9 (69)	24.6 (17)
Cognitive restructuring	47.9 (46)	37.7 (26)
Strategies to deal with hypnotics	33.3 (32)	31.9 (22)
Strategies to deal with stress	33.3 (32)	20.3 (14)
Strategies to deal with daytime symptoms	28.1 (27)	24.6 (17)
Keeping a sleep diary	55.2 (53)	7.2 (5)

Data were collected in a randomized controlled trial of group CBT-I in primary health care[31] and have not been published previously.

personality traits associated with insomnia, such as concerns about making mistakes and setting high personal standards,[33] neuroticism, and conscientiousness,[34] or just unclear PI instructions.

Moreover, the previous study of group CBT-I in primary health care[31] included follow-up questionnaires about the perceived usefulness of each CBT-I component in the intervention (unpublished results). Immediately after therapy, 30.2% (29 of 96) found PI useful and responded that they would use it in the future, and 1 year after therapy, 23.2% (16 of 69) found it useful (**Table 2**). This finding suggests that it could be reasonable to include PI in CBT-I. It should be noted that PI in this study only consisted of one session. A greater dose might render the technique useful for more people.

SUMMARY

This article aimed to review and discuss theoretic and clinical frameworks for PI, the current evidence base for PI, as well as its clinical relevance, and considerations needed when PI is used as an adjunct treatment to CBT-I or as a second-line intervention for insomnia.

The instructions for PI and the rationale given to participants have varied over the years. The most common and prevailing instructions seem to be those described in 1979[2]: "Lie comfortably in bed, in a dark room, with your eyes open. Try to remain awake for as long as possible, without engaging in sleep incompatible activities." The rationale behind these instructions, which is also shared with the patients, is that conscious intent to fall asleep may disturb natural sleep initiation processes, and that PI aims to reduce sleep-related performance anxiety. The rationale is in line with the AIE pathway for the development of insomnia.[8]

PI has been considered an evidence-based treatment by AASM since the 1990s, although PI was not recommended as a single-component treatment in their 2021 clinical practice guidelines for behavioral and psychological treatments for insomnia.[17] It is worth mentioning that the 2021 guidelines were based on a systematic review of 5 trials, and a meta-analysis including 2 trials. However, the previous narrative review of cognitive interventions for insomnia found empirical support for PI,[18] and so did the systematic review and meta-analysis that included 10 trials on PI.[19] In summary, PI can still be considered as an evidence-based treatment that has the potential to reduce sleep onset latency and the number of awakenings. The scientific support for PI refers to PI delivered as a single component treatment. PI has also been included as a cognitive technique in CBT-I, but what PI may add to the outcome results has not been investigated.

Although CBT-I is the treatment of choice, there are issues with a proportion of patients who do not benefit from the treatment, CBT-I might not be suitable for all, and availability varies greatly. It may thus be relevant for clinicians to consider PI as an adjunct intervention for insomnia or as a second-line treatment. The consideration should be based on clinical knowledge and experiences; the circumstances of each patient, including the patient's needs, resources, and preferences; as well as available treatment options. As a treatment, PI should be relatively easy for clinicians to learn, and to deliver in various clinical settings.

According to potential mechanisms of change in PI, it is reasonable to assume that PI may be particularly relevant (as an adjunct- or second-line treatment) for patients with sleep-related performance anxiety and/or sleep-onset insomnia, and that PI will be more successful in patients who have a significant sleep drive because of prolonged wakefulness before going to bed. Moreover, PI may be helpful in reducing sleep-disturbing behaviors in bed and serve as a moment to be aware of anxiety-provoking thoughts.

PI instructions may overlap with those of other CBT-I techniques, which support the use of PI as a second-line intervention. PI may also be contradictory to other CBT-I techniques, which may make it difficult to implement PI as an adjunct intervention in CBT-I. One example is stimulus control, in which the instructions to not engage in sleep-disturbing behaviors is in line with the PI instructions. However, the instructions to get out of bed when unable to fall asleep contrasts with the PI instructions to lie awake in bed as long as possible. Another example is sleep restriction. Sleep restriction means less hours in bed, which aims to reduce wakefulness in bed. There are thus limited opportunities to lie awake for any longer time. On the other hand, sleep restriction will create a significant sleep drive, which may help the patient to fall asleep quickly when using PI, which in turn may help reducing sleep performance anxiety, the main goal of PI.

If PI will be delivered as a second-line, stand-alone treatment, it is currently not possible to recommend a certain dose, but most PI interventions have included 2 to 4 sessions. Negative side effects of PI have not been fully explored, but a side effect to be aware of is, like in other psychological interventions, increased anxiety in the beginning of treatment.

FUTURE RESEARCH

During the writing process of this article, we identified several areas for future research, both on PI as an adjunct treatment of insomnia and as a second-line treatment of insomnia. Most of the previous studies were conducted in the eighties, and we have since seen changes in diagnostic criteria, research methodology, and lifestyle habits (eg, electronic devices).

One area for future research is evaluations of PI in different populations, with a special focus on populations in which CBT-I may be unsuitable, for example, older and frail persons, pregnant women, shift workers, long-distance drivers, patients with bipolar disorder, and patients who do not improve by CBT-I. Moreover, future studies are needed to determine which patients are best suited for PI, for example, patients with sleep-onset insomnia versus sleep-maintenance insomnia. Other areas for future research are to investigate moderators and theory-based mechanisms of change, and the role of PI as an adjunct treatment of insomnia. Moreover, studies on the effects of PI on daytime symptoms and functioning, side effects of PI, and adherence are missing, and so are long-term follow-ups and cost-effectiveness analyses of PI. Inductive explorations of patients' experience of PI are an additional area of research when qualitative studies have the potential to catch experiences that are difficult to catch in by questionnaires and statistical analyses.

CLINICS CARE POINTS

- PI is one of several treatment components that clinicians might consider using as an adjunct intervention to CBT-I.
- As an adjunct intervention, PI could be used after the implementation of CBT-I or concurrently with CBT-I.
- In some cases, PI might be preferred over CBT-I, due to a patient's clinical presentation or the brief nature of PI.

DISCLOSURE

M. Jansson-Fröjmark, C. Sandlund, and A. Norell-Clarke have nothing to disclose.

REFERENCES

1. Ascher LM, Efran JS. Use of paradoxical intention in a behavioral program for sleep onset insomnia. J Consult Clin Psychol 1978;46(3):547–50.
2. Ascher LM, Turner RM. Paradoxical intention and insomnia: an experimental investigation. Behav Res Ther 1979;17(4):408–11.
3. Espie CA. Paradoxical intention therapy. In: Behavioral treatments for sleep disorders. Elsevier; 2011. p. 61–70.

4. Ascher LM, Turner RM. A comparison of two methods for the administration of paradoxical intention. Behav Res Ther 1980;18(2):121–6.

5. Byrne TM. The differential effects of paradoxical intention and relaxation training upon insomnia in depressed and non-depressed subjects. Ann Arbor: Hofstra University; 1983. p. 8410500. ProQuest Dissertations & Theses Global: The Sciences and Engineering Collection database.

6. Fogle DO, Dyal JA. Paradoxical giving up and the reduction of sleep performance anxiety in chronic insomniacs. Psychotherapy: Theor Res Pract 1983; 20(1):21.

7. Ott BD, Levine BA, Ascher LM. Manipulating the explicit demand of paradoxical intention instructions. Behav Cogn Psychotherapy 1983;11(1):25–35.

8. Espie CA, Broomfield NM, MacMahon KMA, et al. The attention-intention-effort pathway in the development of psychophysiologic insomnia: a theoretical review. Sleep Med Rev 2006;10(4):215–45.

9. Harris K, Spiegelhalder K, Espie CA, et al. Sleep-related attentional bias in insomnia: a state-of-the-science review. Clin Psychol Rev 2015;42:16–27.

10. Lundh L-G. Cognitive-behavioural analysis and treatment of insomnia. Scand J Behav Ther 1998; 27(1):10–29.

11. Bothelius K, Jernelöv S, Fredrikson M, et al. Measuring acceptance of sleep difficulties: the development of the sleep problem acceptance questionnaire. Sleep 2015;38(11):1815–22.

12. Ree M, Harvey A. Insomnia. In: Bennett-Levy JE, Butler GE, Fennell ME, editors. Oxford guide to behavioural experiments in cognitive therapy. Oxford: Oxford University Press; 2004. p. 287–305.

13. Salari N, Khazaie H, Hosseinian-Far A, et al. The effect of acceptance and commitment therapy on insomnia and sleep quality: a systematic review. BMC Neurol 2020;20(1):1–18.

14. Morin CM, Hauri PJ, Espie CA, et al. Nonpharmacologic treatment of chronic insomnia. An American Academy of Sleep Medicine review. Sleep 1999; 22(8):1134–56.

15. Morin CM, Bootzin RR, Buysse DJ, et al. Psychological and behavioral treatment of insomnia: update of the recent evidence (1998-2004). Sleep 2006; 29(11):1398–414.

16. Edinger JD, Arnedt JT, Bertisch SM, et al. Behavioral and psychological treatments for chronic insomnia disorder in adults: an American Academy of Sleep Medicine systematic review, meta-analysis, and GRADE assessment. J Clin Sleep Med 2021;17(2): 263–98.

17. Edinger JD, Arnedt JT, Bertisch SM, et al. Behavioral and psychological treatments for chronic insomnia disorder in adults: an American Academy of Sleep Medicine clinical practice guideline. J Clin Sleep Med 2021a;17(2):255–62.

18. Jansson Frojmark M, Norell-Clarke A. The cognitive treatment components and therapies of cognitive behavioral therapy for insomnia: a systematic review. Sleep Med Rev 2018;42:19–36.

19. Jansson-Fröjmark M, Alfonsson S, Bohman B, et al. Paradoxical intention for insomnia: a systematic review and meta-analysis. J Sleep Res 2021;31(2): e13464.

20. Espie CA, Lindsay WR. Paradoxical intention in the treatment of chronic insomnia: six case studies illustrating variability in therapeutic response. Behav Res Ther 1985;23(6):703–9. Retrieved from. http:// www.ncbi.nlm.nih.gov/pubmed/3907617.

21. Kyle SD, Morgan K, Spiegelhalder K, et al. No pain, no gain: an exploratory within-subjects mixed-methods evaluation of the patient experience of sleep restriction therapy (SRT) for insomnia. Sleep Med 2011;12(8):735–47.

22. Craske MG, Treanor M, Conway CC, et al. Maximizing exposure therapy: an inhibitory learning approach. Behav Res Ther 2014;58:10–23.

23. van Straten A, van der Zweerde T, Kleiboer A, et al. Cognitive and behavioral therapies in the treatment of insomnia: a meta-analysis. Sleep Med Rev 2018; 38:3–16.

24. Hasan F, Tu Y-K, Yang C-M, et al. Comparative efficacy of digital cognitive behavioral therapy for insomnia: a systematic review and network meta-analysis. Sleep Med Rev 2022;61:101567.

25. Drerup ML, Ahmed-Jauregui S. Online delivery of cognitive behavioral therapy-insomnia: considerations and controversies. Sleep Med Clin 2019; 14(2):283–90.

26. Sandlund C, Kane K, Ekstedt M, et al. Patients' experiences of motivation, change, and challenges in group treatment for insomnia in primary care: a focus group study. BMC Fam Pract 2018;19(1):1–11.

27. Kyle SD, Miller CB, Rogers Z, et al. Sleep restriction therapy for insomnia is associated with reduced objective total sleep time, increased daytime somnolence, and objectively impaired vigilance: implications for the clinical management of insomnia disorder. Sleep 2014;37(2):229–37.

28. Espie CA, Lindsay WR, Brooks DN, et al. A controlled comparative investigation of psychological treatments for chronic sleep-onset insomnia. Behav Res Ther 1989;27(1):79–88.

29. Riemann D, Baglioni C, Bassetti C, et al. European guideline for the diagnosis and treatment of insomnia. J Sleep Res 2017;26(6). https://doi.org/ 10.1111/jsr.12594.

30. Jansson M, Linton SJ. Cognitive-behavioral group therapy as an early intervention for insomnia: a randomized controlled trial. J Occup Rehabil 2005; 15(2):177–90.

31. Sandlund C, Hetta J, Nilsson GH, et al. Improving insomnia in primary care patients: a randomized

controlled trial of nurse-led group treatment. Int J Nurs Stud 2017;72:30–41.

32. Maurer LF, Espie CA, Omlin X, et al. Isolating the role of time in bed restriction in the treatment of insomnia: a randomized, controlled, dismantling trial comparing sleep restriction therapy with time in bed regularization. Sleep 2020;43(11):zsaa096.

33. Jansson-Fröjmark M, Linton SJ. Is perfectionism related to pre-existing and future insomnia? A prospective study. Br J Clin Psychol 2007;46(1):119–24.

34. Dekker K, Blanken TF, Van Someren EJ. Insomnia and personality—a network approach. Brain Sci 2017;7(3):28.

Circadian Interventions as Adjunctive Therapies to Cognitive-Behavioral Therapy for Insomnia

Leslie M. Swanson, PhD*, Greta B. Raglan, PhD

KEYWORDS

• Circadian • Circadian rhythms • Cognitive-behavioral therapy for insomnia • Insomnia
• Insomnia treatment

KEY POINTS

- The insomnia subtypes of sleep onset insomnia and early morning awakening insomnia are associated with delayed and advanced circadian rhythms, respectively.
- Adjunctive circadian interventions for sleep onset insomnia include morning bright light therapy, scheduled dim light in the evening, and low-dose melatonin administered in the late afternoon/early evening.
- Adjunctive circadian interventions for early-morning awakening insomnia include evening bright light therapy and scheduled dim light in the morning.
- Clinical trials are needed to test adjunctive administration of circadian interventions within a course of cognitive-behavioral therapy for insomnia to inform best practices.

INTRODUCTION

Cognitive-behavioral therapy for insomnia (CBTI) is effective for many individuals who suffer from insomnia; however, a nontrivial proportion of patients who complete treatment will not achieve full remission.[1] Thus, identification of treatment targets for therapies administered adjunctively to CBTI can enhance treatment outcomes. Although attention is paid in CBTI to the role of the circadian system in the pathogenesis of insomnia, the primary therapeutic components are largely focused on behavioral modifications that do not directly target the circadian system. Thus, integrating specific circadian-focused interventions adjunctive to CBTI may enhance treatment outcomes for patients whose insomnia is associated with circadian misalignment.

Circadian rhythms are the 24-hour physiologic and behavioral manifestations of the internal master circadian pacemaker, located in the suprachiasmatic nucleus.[2] Alertness, sleepiness, and the propensity for sleep are key circadian rhythms. Insomnia, a sleep disorder characterized by difficulty falling asleep, staying asleep, and/or early morning awakenings,[3] is linked to dysregulation of circadian rhythms.[4] Although the exact pathophysiology of insomnia remains unknown, evidence implicates the circadian system as an important pathway in the development and maintenance of chronic insomnia.[5,6] For example, a mismatch between the behavioral timing of sleep and the circadian timing of sleepiness/alertness—that is, attempting to sleep at the wrong circadian time—can cause insomnia.[7]

The types of insomnia symptoms reported by the patient can provide clues about whether, and how, circadian rhythms may be contributing to sleep difficulties and aid clinical decision making about whether to integrate a circadian-based therapeutic with CBTI. For example, patients who

Department of Psychiatry, University of Michigan, 4250 Plymouth Road, Ann Arbor, MI 48105, USA
* Corresponding author.
E-mail address: lmswan@med.umich.edu

Sleep Med Clin 18 (2023) 21–30
https://doi.org/10.1016/j.jsmc.2022.09.004
1556-407X/23/

report primarily early morning awakenings and experience sleepiness in the early evening may have a circadian rhythm timed to be abnormally early (circadian phase advance).[8,9] Conversely, patients who report primarily difficulty falling asleep with sleepiness in the morning hours may have a circadian rhythm timed to be abnormally late (circadian phase delay).[10]

This article reviews the role of the circadian system in sleep, circadian dysregulation in insomnia, and practical applications of circadian interventions adjunctive to CBTI, with a focus on bright light therapy, strategically timed dim light and blue-blocking glasses, and exogenous melatonin. It discusses adjunctive circadian-based interventions for patients whose insomnia may be influenced by circadian misalignment as suggested by presentation and clinical interview, but who do not meet full diagnostic criteria for a circadian rhythm sleep-wake disorder. For a more in-depth review of implementation of CBTI in patients who meet full diagnostic criteria for a circadian rhythm sleep-wake disorder, the authors recommend the chapter by Evans and Hasler in Adapting Cognitive Behavioral Therapy for Insomnia.[11]

REGULATION OF SLEEP

The sleep-wake cycle is regulated by the complex interaction between 2 specific systems: the sleep homeostatic system (Process S) and the circadian system (Process C).[12] Briefly, Process S is a homeostatic process whereby the drive for sleep accumulates throughout wakefulness and diminishes during sleep. Process C is determined by the master circadian clock, which produces a circadian rhythm of arousal/sleepiness. The circadian rhythm of arousal/sleepiness across the 24-hour day can be impacted by a variability in the intrinsic circadian period length resulting in a behavioral preference for morning or eveningness (morning larks and night owls, respectively).[13] External zeitgebers (timegivers) also play an important role in entraining the circadian rhythm. The light-dark cycle is the most potent zeitgeber,[14] but other relevant external inputs to the circadian clock include social activity, feeding, and physical activity.[15,16] Markers of the timing of process C include core body temperature and melatonin rhythms; falling body temperature and rising melatonin levels herald sleep, whereas rising body temperature and falling melatonin levels presage wake.[17] To sleep well, the behavioral timing of sleep must be aligned with Process C and Process S—that is, sleep is attempted when both the homeostatic drive for sleep and circadian rhythm of sleepiness are high.

Sleep is inhibited by Process C at specific times, even when the homeostatic drive (Process S) for sleep may be high, via an alerting signal. A 2- to 3-hour forbidden zone for sleep occurs in the early evening (about 1 to 4 hours before habitual sleep onset time); the propensity for sleep is low at this time.[18] For someone who typically falls asleep around 11 p.m., the forbidden zone for sleep would occur from 6 to 9 p.m. In the morning, a wake-up zone facilitates awakening, approximately between 8 and 11 a.m. for someone who goes to bed around 11 p.m.[18] These zones hold particular relevance for insomnia; an individual who has delayed (ie, late) circadian timing but attempts to sleep during the forbidden zone will have difficulty falling asleep. An individual who has advanced (ie, early) circadian timing but attempts to sleep through the wake-up zone will have difficulty with sleep maintenance/early awakening.

CIRCADIAN DYSREGULATION IN INSOMNIA
Sleep-Onset Insomnia

Difficulty falling asleep accompanied by morning sleepiness/fatigue, in the absence of difficulty with sleep maintenance and early morning awakenings, may indicate a subtype of insomnia—sleep-onset insomnia—linked to a delayed circadian rhythm. This type of insomnia is often observed in younger adults who have difficulty sleeping on a schedule dictated by their work/social obligations. Adults with sleep-onset insomnia have a later time of melatonin onset compared to adults without insomnia.[10,19–21] An investigation of sleep and circadian timing in adults with insomnia revealed that adults with insomnia attempted to fall asleep at the same clock time as good-sleeping controls, but their circadian clocks were delayed by more than 1 hour on average.[10] More specifically, in this study, good-sleeping controls attempted to fall asleep 3 hours and 10 minutes after their melatonin onset occurred, whereas participants with insomnia went to bed 2 hours 13 minutes after melatonin onset; the patients with insomnia were trying to fall asleep during their forbidden zone, during which sleep onset latency will be prolonged.[10] Sleeping in on the weekends (ie, a later wake time on the weekends relative to weekdays) can cause a circadian phase delay and contribute to an increased length of time to fall asleep at the start of the week.[22]

Early Morning Awakening Insomnia

Insomnia characterized by waking up too early with an inability to resume sleep and sleepiness/

fatigue in the early evening, in the absence of difficulty falling asleep, may indicate a subtype of insomnia—early morning awakening insomnia—linked to an advanced circadian rhythm. This type of insomnia is most frequently observed in older adults who may report that they inadvertently doze off or fall asleep on the couch or recliner in the early evening and subsequently wake up too early in the morning. Compared with good sleepers, adults with early morning awakening insomnia have significantly earlier circadian timing as indicated by earlier body temperature and melatonin rhythms.[9,18] Their sleep period is also timed such that a considerable portion overlaps with the wake-up zone.[9]

APPLYING CIRCADIAN INTERVENTIONS ADJUNCTIVE TO COGNITIVE-BEHAVIORAL THERAPY FOR INSOMNIA

Interventions that target the circadian system and are most readily adjunctively administered to CBTI include strategically timed bright light, strategically timed dim light, and melatonin (**Table 1**). Here the authors briefly discuss relevant physiology for each intervention while maintaining a focus on clinical implementation. For a thorough overview of the impact of light and melatonin on human circadian physiology, the reader is referred to Emens and Burgess.[23]

The specific implementation of each intervention depends on the patient's insomnia subtype. An important caveat to circadian-based interventions is that if the interventions are not timed correctly, they may actually worsen the patient's sleep. Thus, careful attention to the patient's sleep timing and the timing of the interventions is important; **Fig. 1** summarizes the timing for each intervention relative to the sleep period by insomnia subtype.

Although the authors outline suggestions for when to begin each circadian intervention relative to the first session of CBTI to maximize efficacy, there are no contraindications to adjunctive administration of CBTI. Some elements of CBTI (ie, strict time in bed scheduling with maintenance of a consistent wake time throughout treatment) will enhance implementation of the circadian interventions. Indeed, time in bed restriction may help to realign the behavioral timing of sleep and the circadian propensity for sleep. Specifically, in a small study of adults with insomnia, after 2 weeks of sleep restriction therapy (ie, time in bed restriction) patients attempted sleep later, while their circadian timing remained the same—meaning they attempted sleep at a more appropriate circadian time.[24]

Strategically Timed Bright Light Exposure

As the most potent zeitgeber,[14] strategically timed bright light exposure is a powerful tool to help patients move their circadian rhythms earlier or later to realign their circadian timing with their desired sleep time. A recent meta-analysis supports the role of light therapy for treatment of insomnia, although it is important to note that the number of studies focused specifically on patients with insomnia are limited, and effect sizes were relatively small, confirming its utility as an adjunctive, but not stand-alone, insomnia therapy.[25] Importantly, light intensity mediated treatment outcomes in this meta-analysis, such that larger treatment effects were observed in studies using brighter light (ie, higher lux).[25]

The impact of light therapy on circadian timing depends on the time at which light therapy is administered, described in a phase response curve to light (**Fig. 2**).[26] As shown in the phase response curve, exposure to bright light in the

---

Table 1
Summary of circadian interventions by insomnia subtype

		Circadian Intervention		
	Bright Light: Intensity	**Bright Light: Dose and Timing**	**Dim Light AND/OR Blue-Blocking Glasses**	**Melatonin**
Sleep onset insomnia	10,000 lux light box OR light glasses	30–60 min at scheduled wake time	90–120 min before scheduled bedtime	0.5 mg taken 5 h before habitual sleep onset time
Early morning awakening insomnia	2500 lux light box	In evening, ending between 0–3 h before scheduled bedtime	From bedtime through 1 h after scheduled wake time	Not indicated

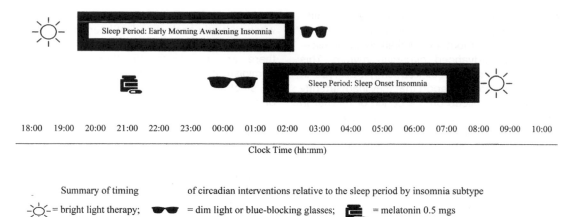

Summary of timing   of circadian interventions relative to the sleep period by insomnia subtype

-☀- = bright light therapy;   🕶 = dim light or blue-blocking glasses;   📱 = melatonin 0.5 mgs

Fig. 1. Summary of timing of circadian interventions relative to the sleep period by insomnia subtype = bright light therapy; dim light or blue-blocking glasses; melatonin 0.5 mg.

hours before habitual sleep onset (starting about 4 hours before) will delay (move later) circadian phase. Conversely, exposure to bright light in the morning (starting about 2 hours before habitual wake time) will advance (move earlier) circadian phase. Note that if morning light is timed too early (that is, more than 2 hours before habitual wake time), it can exacerbate a circadian phase delay and lead to lengthening of the sleep onset.

Bright Light Therapy Considerations

Device selection

Various light therapy devices are commercially available, and guidance should be provided to patients regarding the specific features to assist them in selecting an effective device. Historically, light therapy was delivered by light boxes. More recently, wearable devices (eg, light therapy glasses) have emerged as an effective treatment option[27-29] with the distinct advantages of mobility and portability. The circadian system is most sensitive to blue-green light (wavelength between 470 to 525 nm[30-32]), and devices that emit light in this wavelength can offer effective therapy at dimmer settings than broad-spectrum light; wearable devices often use light in this wavelength.[33] An ideal wearable device will project light upwards from below the eye, so the supraorbital ridge does not block the light.

Patients interested in a light box should look for a broad-spectrum or blue-green light-emitting box that emits between 2500 and 10,000 lux; patients with early morning awakening insomnia may find benefit on the lower end of this range (ie, 2500 lux), whereas patients with sleep-onset insomnia should look for a box with higher lux (ie, 10,000 lux). Patients who use a light box can be instructed to measure and cut an appropriate length of string

(typically 2 feet) to be taped to the box to make sure they are sitting at the correct distance from the box.[23] In their clinical practice, the authors have found that wearable light therapy glasses offer the most practical way for patients to receive bright light therapy, as they can carry out much of their morning routine and engage in activities such as watching television, or working on a computer or tablet, while receiving effective therapy.

Side effects and contraindications

The most common side effects of bright light therapy are headache, eyestrain, nausea, and agitation, but these often spontaneously remit within 1 to 2 weeks of use.[34,35] The dose can be adjusted (eg, reduced to 30 or even 15 minutes) as needed to address side effects. Contraindications for bright light therapy include certain medical conditions (eg, epilepsy/seizure, lupus or other medical conditions associated with photosensitivity, retinal pathology, or retinal surgery) and use of photosensitizing medications. Individuals with a history of mania/hypomania or bipolar disorder may use light therapy but must be closely monitored to prevent possible recurrence of mania/hypomania triggered by overexposure to light, which is rare but serious should it occur.[35] In their clinical experience, the authors have found that bright light therapy for insomnia is typically well-tolerated without significant side effects or adverse events.

Bright Light Therapy for Sleep-Onset Insomnia

Incorrectly timed bright light therapy can worsen a circadian phase delay and exacerbate difficulty falling asleep. When integrating light therapy with CBTI, patients should maintain a consistent wake time throughout the course of therapy. The authors

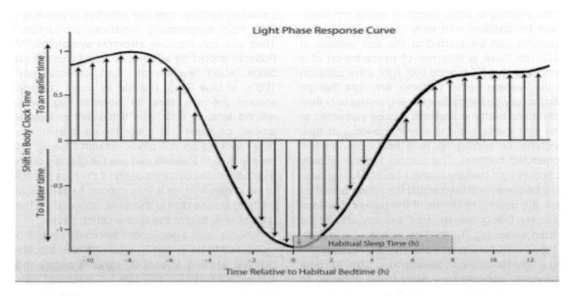

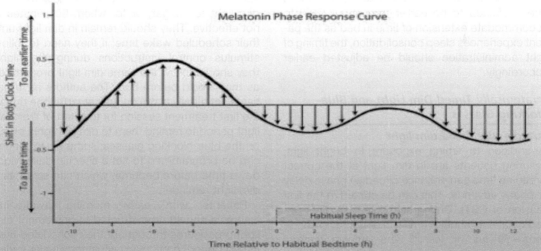

Fig. 2. Phase response curves to light and melatonin. (*From* Emens JS, Burgess HJ. Effect of light and melatonin and other melatonin receptor agonists on human circadian physiology. Sleep Med Clin 2015;10(4):435-453; with permission.)

recommend waiting to initiate light therapy until the second CBTI treatment session, generally only after the patient has maintained a consistent wake time across both weekdays and weekends, and physicians are confident in the patient's ability to continue this; sleeping in on the weekends can contribute to light therapy overlapping with the phase delay portion of the phase response curve on weekdays. Emphasizing the importance of maintaining a consistent wake time, even on weekends, when undergoing morning light therapy, and providing the rationale for this instruction, can enhance the patient's adherence.

Once the patient is ready to begin light therapy, he or she should be instructed to use light therapy device for 30 to 60 minutes as close to their scheduled wake time as possible, ideally starting no later than 30 minutes after their scheduled wake time. Patients should be instructed to delay starting light therapy until their scheduled wake time if they wake earlier. The length of treatment may depend on what the patient's morning schedule allows; although 60 minutes will elicit a more robust treatment response, 30 minutes is often more pragmatic and sufficient to improve sleep.[36,37]

Bright light therapy for early morning awakening insomnia
Patients whose insomnia is primarily characterized by early morning awakenings can use light therapy

in the evening to delay circadian timing.[8,38] Treatment for patients with early morning awakening insomnia can be started at the first session of CBTI, as there is little risk of exacerbation of a circadian phase advance with light administration in the evening before bedtime, and light therapy can assist with the patient staying awake until their scheduled bedtime. Patients can be instructed to use light therapy in the evening, ending at their bedtime, or ending up to 3 hours before their scheduled bedtime. The authors typically initially schedule light therapy to end 1 hour before scheduled bedtime, and then adjust the timing based on how the patient responds. If the patient develops difficulty falling asleep, light therapy should be ended earlier (eg, 1.5 to 3 hours before bedtime). If they report persistence of early morning awakenings, light therapy can be extended later. In some instances, patients may need to be exposed to bright light right until their bedtime. As bedtime is often adjusted to be earlier throughout CBTI to accommodate extension of time in bed as the patient experiences sleep consolidation, the timing of light administration should be adjusted earlier accordingly.

Strategically Timed Dim Light and Blue-Blocking Glasses

Strategically timed dim light
In addition to timing exposure to bright light, ensuring patients are in dim light at the correct circadian time can enhance circadian phase delay or phase advance. This can be started in the first session of CBTI. During scheduled dim light periods, patients should remain in dim lighting conditions—50 lux or less.[39] The authors instruct patients to use just enough light to see during their scheduled dim light period; ideally, light-emitting devices (smartphones, tablets, computer screens) would not be used during time.[40] Depending on the time of year and the patient's latitude, patients may have to employ light-blocking curtains or window coverings to minimize exposure to sunlight during the dim light period. Patients may watch television on an actual television set during this time, ideally with all other light sources turned off.[41] Patients who find it necessary to use a light-emitting device (eg, smartphone, tablet, computer) during their dim light period may use the device, provided the device is dimmed to the lowest possible setting, or the patient can wear blue-blocking glasses.[40]

Blue-blocking glasses
Blue-blocking glasses filter out blue-green wavelength light and therefore limit ocular exposure to wavelengths of light most impactful to the circadian system; they are effective in preventing light from suppressing melatonin production.[42] Their use can improve insomnia symptoms.[43,44] Patients should be advised to select glasses that block short wavelength light (approximately 100% of blue light), provide as much coverage around the eye area as possible (eg, wraparound lenses), and have tinted lenses (orange, amber, or brown), as clear lenses marketed as blue-blocking do not block enough blue light to be effective.[45] Patients can use the glasses during their scheduled dim light period if they are not able to be in dim light, or if they choose to use a light-emitting device during this time, especially if they are not able to dim the light-emitting device.

Patients with sleep-onset insomnia should be instructed to be in dim light (or use blue-blocking glasses) starting a least 90 minutes before their scheduled bedtime; this can be extended up to 120 minutes for patients who are able to be in dim light for longer, or for whom 90 minutes is not effective. They should remain in dim light until their scheduled wake time; if they need to follow stimulus control instructions during the night, they should follow the same dim light procedures as they would before bed. The authors have patients set a daily alarm on their smartphone during the first treatment session for the start of their dim light period to remind them to dim the lights or put on the blue-blocking glasses; some smartphones can be programmed to set a specific daily wind-down time before bedtime, which can serve as a dim light reminder.

Patients with early morning awakening insomnia should be instructed to implement dim light procedures throughout their scheduled time in bed period, particularly when they wake earlier than their scheduled wake time (ie, remain in dim light until their wake-up alarm) to avoid potentially exacerbating their early morning awakenings with morning light exposure. Ideally, patients with this type of insomnia would also avoid bright light exposure for the first hour after their scheduled wake time when possible. Strategies to facilitate this include wearing dark sunglasses if patients must be outdoors (eg, commuting to work) within an hour of their scheduled wake time, and avoiding light-emitting devices during this time. Blue-blocking glasses can be worn as needed. In some instances, patients with early morning awakening insomnia require a more limited dim light period before bedtime (dim light starting less than 60 minutes before bedtime), or they should avoid a dim light period before bed altogether, particularly if they are inadvertently falling asleep during the dim light procedures before bedtime.

Exogeneous Melatonin

Exogenous melatonin, an over-the-counter supplement, can be helpful in reducing sleep onset latency in insomnia but is not likely to be beneficial for sleep maintenance or early morning awakenings.[46–48] Melatonin can be used as a both hypnotic and as a zeitgeber.[49] The authors focus on its use as a zeitgeber to advance circadian phase. As a zeitgeber, melatonin has its own phase response curve (see **Fig. 2**); administration in the late afternoon until about 2 hours before habitual sleep onset time will advance circadian phase, whereas administration timed within 2 hours of habitual sleep onset time through the morning hours will delay circadian phase.[50,51] As with the light response curve, this means that taking melatonin at the wrong time (too close to habitual sleep onset time) can exacerbate a circadian phase delay.

It is important to tell patients that the dosing instructions for melatonin found on the bottle (indicating that the patient should take it 30 to 60 minutes before bed) are for use of melatonin as a soporific and should be disregarded. Patients who have difficulty falling asleep and are interested in using melatonin as adjunctive to CBTI should be instructed to use a small dose (0.5 mg) of melatonin taken 5 hours before their typical sleep onset time. The authors prefer use of a small dose of melatonin (0.5 mg) based on work showing similar phase shifting effects between smaller (0.3 to 0.5 mg) and larger (3.0 mg) doses to maximize efficacy while minimizing soporific effects and the possibility of overlap with the phase delay portion of the phase response curve.[51,52] As 0.5 mg of melatonin may not be commercially available, the authors tell patients to purchase 1 mg tablets and cut them in half. During the treatment session, the authors have patients set a daily alarm on their smartphone for their scheduled melatonin administration time, as many forget to take melatonin at the desired time without the reminder alarm. Melatonin may be used in conjunction with bright light therapy for sleep-onset insomnia; the combination may enhance circadian phase advances.[53]

Side effects and contraindications for melatonin

Melatonin is not regulated by the US Food and Drug Administration, and the actual melatonin content in the tablet may vary from the label on the bottle.[54] Although extended-release formulations are available, the authors do not recommend them, as they may lead spillover of melatonin into the phase delay period.[55] Although melatonin is widely used and available over-the-counter, it may cause side effects and negatively interact with frequently used medications and common medical conditions (see https://naturalmedicines.therapeuticresearch.com for a comprehensive list of possible interactions and possible side effects). The most common side effects of melatonin include drowsiness, headache, dizziness, and nausea.[56] Because of the potential for drowsiness, patients should not use alcohol, or operate a motor vehicle or heavy machinery while taking melatonin until they know how they respond to low-dose afternoon melatonin. Relative contraindications for melatonin include diabetes, hypertension, clotting/bleeding disorders (including warfarin therapy), seizures/epilepsy, pregnancy/attempting conception, and breastfeeding because of interactions with these conditions, drugs used to treat these conditions, and an unknown safety profile for fetuses and in breastfeeding.[56] Melatonin may interact with many prescription medications, supplements, and medical conditions. The most commonly used medications that may interact with melatonin include antihypertensives, immunosuppressants, antidiabetes drugs, and anticoagulant/antiplatelet medications.[57] Although melatonin may reduce blood pressure in healthy individuals, it may increase blood pressure in patients taking antihypertensive medications, and it reduces the effectiveness of some antihypotensive medications in animal studies.[57] Caution is recommended when taking melatonin in combination with antidiabetes drugs because of some evidence that suggests that melatonin may impair glucose metabolism.[57] Melatonin may interfere with immunosuppressive therapy by stimulating immune function, increase the risk of seizure activity when taken with drugs that lower the seizure threshold, and have antiplatelet effects that increase the risk of bleeding with anticoagulant/antiplatelet therapies.[57] Moreover, melatonin has only been studied in short-term trials; larger-scale randomized controlled trials of longer duration are needed to establish the long-term safety of melatonin.

SUMMARY

The circadian system plays an important role in the regulation of the sleep-wake cycle. Dysregulation of circadian rhythms, or misalignment between the behavioral timing of sleep and the circadian propensity for sleep, can contribute to the development and maintenance of insomnia, even in the absence of a frank circadian rhythm sleep-wake disorder. Patients who present with specific subtypes of insomnia (ie, sleep-onset insomnia or early morning awakening insomnia) most closely linked to circadian rhythm dysregulation may benefit from circadian interventions administered adjunctively to CBTI. Specific interventions to consider include bright light therapy, strategically timed dim light, and exogenous melatonin. However, careful attention must be paid to the timing of these interventions to ensure their success. Further, although overall evidence supports the use of these interventions in insomnia, there is a need for trials testing adjunctive administration of circadian interventions within a course of CBTI to determine best practices for implementation.

CLINICS CARE POINTS

- Patients who present with sleep-onset insomnia may be prescribed bright light therapy in the morning in conjunction with dim light in the evening before bed to aid in advancing circadian phase.

- A small dose (0.5 mg) of melatonin taken in the late afternoon (approximately 5 hours before habitual sleep onset time) may help advance circadian phase in patients who have sleep-onset insomnia.

- Bright light in the evening before bedtime in conjunction with dim light for 1 hour after scheduled wake-up time may improve sleep in patients with early morning awakenings by delaying their circadian phase.

- Blue-blocking glasses can improve insomnia by reducing light exposure during scheduled dim light periods.

DISCLOSURE

The authors have no disclosures or conflicts of interest to report.

REFERENCES

1. Brasure M, Fuchs E, MacDonald R, et al. Psychological and behavioral interventions for managing insomnia disorder: an evidence report for a clinical practice guideline by the American College of Physicians. Ann Intern Med 2016;165(2):113–24.
2. Moore RY. Organization and function of a central nervous system circadian oscillator: the suprachiasmatic hypothalamic nucleus. Fed Proc 1983;42(11): 2783–9.
3. Ford ES, Cunningham TJ, Giles WH, et al. Trends in insomnia and excessive daytime sleepiness among U.S. adults from 2002 to 2012. Sleep Med 2015; 16(3):372–8.
4. American Academy of Sleep Medicine. International classification of sleep disorders. 3rd edition. Darien, IL: American Academy of Sleep Medicine; 2014.
5. Levenson JC, Kay DB, Buysse DJ. The pathophysiology of insomnia. Chest 2015;147(4):1179–92.
6. Lack LC, Gradisar M, Van Someren EJ, et al. The relationship between insomnia and body temperatures. Sleep Med Rev 2008;12(4):307–17.
7. Dijk DJ, Czeisler CA. Paradoxical timing of the circadian rhythm of sleep propensity serves to consolidate sleep and wakefulness in humans. Neurosci Lett 1994;166(1):63–8.
8. Lack L, Wright H. The effect of evening bright light in delaying the circadian rhythms and lengthening the sleep of early morning awakening insomniacs. Sleep 1993;16(5):436–43.
9. Lack LC, Mercer JD, Wright H. Circadian rhythms of early morning awakening insomniacs. J Sleep Res 1996;5(4):211–9.
10. Flynn-Evans EE, Shekleton JA, Miller B, et al. Circadian phase and phase angle disorders in primary insomnia. Sleep 2017;40(12). https://doi.org/10.1093/sleep/zsx163.
11. Evans MA, Hasler BP. CBT-I for patients with phase disorders or insomnia with circadian misalignment. In: Nowakowski S, Garland SN, Grandner MA, et al, editors. Adapting cognitive behavioral therapy for insomnia. Academic Press; 2022. p. 63–95.
12. Borbély AA, Daan S, Wirz-Justice A, et al. The two-process model of sleep regulation: a reappraisal. J Sleep Res 2016;25(2):131–43.
13. Duffy JF, Rimmer DW, Czeisler CA. Association of intrinsic circadian period with morningness-eveningness, usual wake time, and circadian phase. Behav Neurosci 2001;115(4):895–9.
14. Czeisler CA, Allan JS, Strogatz SH, et al. Bright light resets the human circadian pacemaker independent of the timing of the sleep-wake cycle. Science 1986; 233:667–71.
15. Quante M, Mariani S, Weng J, et al. Zeitgebers and their association with rest-activity patterns. Chronobiol 2019;36(2):203–13.
16. Mistlberger RE, Skene DJ. Nonphotic entrainment in humans? J Biol Rhythms 2005;20(4):339–52.
17. Benloucif S, Guico MJ, Reid KJ, et al. Stability of melatonin and temperature as circadian phase markers and their relationship to sleep times in humans. J Biol Rhythms 2005;20(2):178–88.
18. Strogatz SH, Kronauer RE, Czeisler CA. Circadian pacemaker interferes with sleep onset at specific times each day: role in insomnia. Am J Physiol 1987;253(1 Pt 2):R172–8.
19. Van Veen MM, Kooij JJ, Boonstra AM, et al. Delayed circadian rhythm in adults with attention-deficit/hyperactivity disorder and chronic sleep-onset insomnia. Biol Psychiatry 2010;67(11):1091–6.

20. Rodenbeck A, Huether G, Rüther E, et al. Altered circadian melatonin secretion patterns in relation to sleep in patients with chronic sleep-wake rhythm disorders. J Pineal Res 1998;25(4):201–10.

21. Wright HR, Lack L, Bootzin RR. Relationship between dim light melatonin onset and the timing of sleep in sleep onset insomniacs. Sleep Biol Rhythms 2006;4:78–80.

22. Taylor A, Wright HR, Lack LC. Sleeping-in on the weekend delays circadian phase and increases sleepiness the following week. Sleep Biol Rhythms 2008;6(3):172–9.

23. Emens JS, Burgess HJ. Effect of light and melatonin and other melatonin receptor agonists on human circadian physiology. Sleep Med Clin 2015;10(4):435–53.

24. Maurer LF, Ftouni S, Espie CA, et al. The acute effects of sleep restriction therapy for insomnia on circadian timing and vigilance. J Sleep Res 2021;30(4):e13260.

25. van Maanen A, Meijer AM, van der Heijden KB, et al. The effects of light therapy on sleep problems: a systematic review and meta-analysis. Sleep Med Rev 2016;29:52–62.

26. St Hilaire MA, Gooley JJ, Khalsa SB, et al. Human phase response curve to a 1 h pulse of bright white light. J Physiol 2012;590(13):3035–45.

27. Hasler B, Buysse D, Ngari W, et al. Successful sleep extension and phase advance in adolescents in response to a pilot sleep/circadian manipulation. Sleep 2019;42:A329–30.

28. Lau T, Lovato N, Lack L. Evaluation of a portable light device for phase advancing the circadian rhythm in the home environment. Sleep Biol Rhythms 2018;16(4):405–11.

29. Lovato N, Lack L. Circadian phase delay using the newly developed re-timer portable light device. Sleep Biol Rhythm 2016;14(2):157–64.

30. Gooley JJ, Lu J, Chou TC, et al. Melanopsin in cells of origin of the retinohypothalamic tract. Nat Neurosci 2001;4(12):1165.

31. LeGates TA, Fernandez DC, Hattar S. Light as a central modulator of circadian rhythms, sleep and affect. Nat Rev Neurosci 2014;15(7):443–54.

32. Wright HR, Lack LC, Kennaway DJ. Differential effects of light wavelength in phase advancing the melatonin rhythm. J Pineal Res Mar 2004;36(2):140–4.

33. Mottram V, Middleton B, Williams P, et al. The impact of bright artificial white and 'blue-enriched' light on sleep and circadian phase during the polar winter. J Sleep Res 2011;20(1 Pt 2):154–61.

34. Pail G, Huf W, Pjrek E, et al. Bright-light therapy in the treatment of mood disorders. Neuropsychobiology 2011;64(3):152–62.

35. Terman M, Terman JS. Light therapy for seasonal and nonseasonal depression: efficacy, protocol, safety, and side effects. CNS Spectr 2005;10(8):647–63 [quiz: 672].

36. Eastman CI, Young MA, Fogg LF, et al. Bright light treatment of winter depression: a placebo-controlled trial. Arch Gen Psychiatry 1998;55(10):883–9.

37. Burgess HJ, Fogg LF, Young MA, et al. Bright light therapy for winter depression–is phase advancing beneficial? Chronobiol 2004;21(4–5):759–75.

38. Duffy JF, Czeisler CA. Effect of light on human circadian physiology. Sleep Med Clin 2009;4(2):165–77.

39. Zeitzer JM, Dijk DJ, Kronauer R, et al. Sensitivity of the human circadian pacemaker to nocturnal light: melatonin phase resetting and suppression. J Physiol 2000;526(Pt 3):695–702.

40. Wood B, Rea MS, Plitnick B, et al. Light level and duration of exposure determine the impact of self-luminous tablets on melatonin suppression. Appl Ergon 2013;44(2):237–40.

41. Figueiro MG, Wood B, Plitnick B, et al. The impact of watching television on evening melatonin levels. J Soc Inf Disp 2013;21(10):417–21.

42. Sasseville A, Paquet N, Sévigny J, et al. Blue blocker glasses impede the capacity of bright light to suppress melatonin production. J Pineal Res 2006;41(1):73–8.

43. Shechter A, Kim EW, St-Onge MP, et al. Blocking nocturnal blue light for insomnia: a randomized controlled trial. J Psychiatr Res 2018;96:196–202.

44. Hester L, Dang D, Barker CJ, et al. Evening wear of blue-blocking glasses for sleep and mood disorders: a systematic review. Chronobiol 2021;38(10):1375–83.

45. Shechter A, Quispe KA, Mizhquiri Barbecho JS, et al. Interventions to reduce short-wavelength ("blue") light exposure at night and their effects on sleep: a systematic review and meta-analysis. Sleep Adv 2020;1(1). https://doi.org/10.1093/sleepadvances/zpaa002.

46. Baglioni C, Bostanova Z, Bacaro V, et al. A systematic review and network meta-analysis of randomized controlled trials evaluating the evidence base of melatonin, light exposure, exercise, and complementary and alternative medicine for patients with insomnia disorder. J Clin Med 2020;9(6):1949.

47. Low TL, Choo FN, Tan SM. The efficacy of melatonin and melatonin agonists in insomnia - an umbrella review. J Psychiatr Res 2020;121:10–23.

48. Auld F, Maschauer EL, Morrison I, et al. Evidence for the efficacy of melatonin in the treatment of primary adult sleep disorders. Sleep Med Rev 2017;34:10–22.

49. Wirz-Justice A, Benedetti F, Terman M. Chronotherapeutics for affective disorders: a clinician's manual

for light and wake therapy. Basel, Switzerland: Karger; 2009.

50. Burgess HJ, Revell VL, Eastman CI. A three pulse phase response curve to three milligrams of melatonin in humans. J Physiol 2008;586(2):639–47.

51. Burgess HJ, Revell VL, Molina TA, et al. Human phase response curves to three days of daily melatonin: 0.5 mg versus 3.0 mg. J Clin Endocrinol Metab 2010;95(7):3325–31.

52. Mundey K, Benloucif S, Harsanyi K, et al. Phase-dependent treatment of delayed sleep phase syndrome with melatonin. Sleep 2005;28(10):1271–8.

53. Paul MA, Gray GW, Lieberman HR, et al. Phase advance with separate and combined melatonin and light treatment. Psychopharmacology 2011; 214(2):515–23.

54. Erland LAE, Saxena PK. Melatonin natural health products and supplements: presence of serotonin and significant variability of melatonin content. J Clin Sleep Med 2017;13(02):275–81.

55. Lewy AJ, Emens J, Jackman A, et al. Circadian uses of melatonin in humans. Chronobiol 2006;23(1–2):403–12.

56. Andersen LP, Gogenur I, Rosenberg J, et al. The safety of melatonin in humans. Clin Drug Investig 2016;36(3):169–75.

57. Melatonin. Food, herbs & supplements. In: Natural medicines [internet database]. Somerville, MA: Therapeutic Research Center; 2022. Available at: https://naturalmedicines.therapeuticresearch.com/databases/food-herbs-supplements.aspx. Accessed March 18, 2022.

Behavioral Activation as an Adjunct Treatment to CBT-I

Jeffrey Young, PHD, CBSM, DBSM

KEYWORDS

• Insomnia • Behavioral • Activation • Sleep

KEY POINTS

- Behavioral activation (BA) is generally recognized as having been integrated into the standard CBT-I approach. However, little research exists that addresses the independent contribution of BA to overall treatment outcome.
- BA, itself, is an empirically validated and robust treatment for depression and there is evidence that BA can decrease insomnia severity in an insomnia comorbid with depression sample.
- Insomnia and depression are commonly comorbid and are related bidirectionally suggesting that there may be a factor among them that could serve as a common target for treatment.

INTRODUCTION

This issue is dedicated to exploring the utility of various adjunctive and alternate interventions in the treatment of insomnia. In this section, behavioral activation (BA) is examined and discussed as an adjunct intervention. As such, it is assumed that BA is being incorporated into well-established and empirically validated treatment protocols such as CBT-I[1–3] or supported by core behavioral components such as stimulus control (SC)[4] and sleep restriction (SR).[5]

WHAT IS BEHAVIORAL ACTIVATION?

Quite commonly, when patients suffer psychologically, they may, in response, withdraw from or avoid previously rewarding activities as those activities may now serve as a trigger for emotional pain. Withdrawal from an emotionally painful experience is maintained by negative reinforcement via a temporary reduction in distress: consider the initial relief when a dreaded social obligation is canceled. However, most often, this withdrawal only serves to perpetuate the very suffering that the patient wishes to purge from their life. BA is a psychotherapeutic technique that can be used as a counterbalance to this kind of maladaptation.

At its core, BA is a psychotherapy formulated to help patients identify behaviors that enhance well-being and psychological health. Further, BA also provides the support structure to help patients maintain those behaviors in the face of psychological resistance, distress, and demoralization. For example, a prescribed morning rise time can be quite challenging for someone who is depressed and sleep deprived. Add in a level of sleep inertia and circadian mismatch and the pull to stay in bed becomes that much stronger. Despite being of value to the patient, getting out of bed will take considerable effort as every fiber in that person protests to stay put. However, with proper psychological support, the patient makes it out of bed. Soon after, the sensorium begins to clear. Sunlight and a morning meal are taken—mood may improve. Overall, what ensues is an enhanced sense of self-efficacy and agency which forms the basis for *out-of-bed at prescribed time* to increase in frequency via positive reinforcement.

University of California, Los Angeles, Semel Institute of Neuroscience and Human Behavior, 300 UCLA Medical Plaza, Suite 1200, Los Angeles, CA 90095, USA
E-mail address: j.young@ucla.edu

Sleep Med Clin 18 (2023) 31–38
https://doi.org/10.1016/j.jsmc.2022.10.002
1556-407X/23/

IDENTIFY BEHAVIORS *AND* THE VALUES THAT SUPPORT THOSE BEHAVIORS

A central tenet of BA is that the behaviors identified should closely correspond not only to a patient's goals but also their values. Values direct a person toward behaving in accordance with what is most important and are distinguished from goals which are, in the end, only achieved or not achieved.[6] That is, one can continuously act in accordance with one's values independent of a discrete goal having been achieved. Taking this kind of value-based approach allows for an expanded repertoire of behaviors that are subject to positive reinforcement because it is now not only the achievement of a goal but also the good-faith effort in service of that achievement that has potency as a reinforcer.

EXAMPLE OF GOALS AND SUPPORTING VALUES

Goal: Leave bed and bedroom at first sign of frustration while lying awake.

Value: "Improving my sleep is important and I can do this by reducing conditioned arousal."

Behavior: "Got out of bed and bedroom only about 50% of the time. Sometimes, it was just too hard to get out of bed in the middle of the night."

Outcome: Here, the stated goal was achieved only in part, whereas the value was upheld.

EMPIRICAL SUPPORT FOR BEHAVIORAL ACTIVATION FOR DEPRESSION

Advancing the understanding of the functional relationship between behavior and depression, and how this relationship informs the treatment for depression has been the primary focus of BA from its inception.[7,8] Over the succeeding years, BA has developed into a well-established, empirically validated, and highly effective treatment for depression.[9–13] Of note, there is evidence that supports BA as being equal in efficacy to cognitive therapy and antidepressant medication[11] and evidence to support BA as being efficacious when deployed either as a monotherapy or in conjunction with cognitive components such as cognitive restructuring.[9,10,14]

EMPIRICAL SUPPORT FOR BEHAVIORAL ACTIVATION FOR INSOMNIA

At present, there is little empirical research that examines the *independent effects* of BA on insomnia, either in the context of a formal insomnia diagnosis[15,16] or in the context of BAs effect on general sleep health and quality. In addition, there seems to be no studies that have attempted to dismantle the effects CBT-I with the purpose of isolating the independent contribution of BA to treatment outcome. This does not translate to suggest that empirically supported applications of BA are not part of the treatment of insomnia as it stands. It is understood that the elements of BA are present in CBT-I, if only incidentally. Further, approaches such as Behavioral Activation and Behavioral Insomnia Therapy (BABIT) and RISE-UP are examples of approaches that incorporate BA, and their application will be discussed in detail later.

To the best of the author's knowledge, the only studies that have approached isolating the role of BA in the treatment of insomnia are those conducted by Yi[17] and Lin and colleagues.[18] Yi examined how BA might be used to improve both sleep and general quality of life in Chinese family members tasked with providing care for a family member with dementia. This pilot study was conducted in two phases. The aim of the first phase was to develop the specific BA protocol, informed by existing literature and qualitative information gathered from interviews of the caregivers. From this, an eight-session telephone-based intervention was developed. The aim of the second phase of the study was to test the efficacy of the newly developed intervention. A total of 71 family caregivers participated. Thirty-five subjects were randomized to the BA intervention and thirty-six subjects were randomized to the control group. Although the clinical significance may be arguably weak, Yi found that the BA intervention yielded significant differences between the intervention and control group as measured by the Pittsburgh Sleep Quality Index Chinese Version (CPSQI) Global score and by the Sleep Quality sub-score of the CPSQI. These results provide a measure of support for the use of BA in insomnia but should be considered tentative and in need of replication.

Lin and colleagues[18] evaluated treatment outcome using either CBT-I or Behavioral Activation for Depression (BAT-D) in patients with co-morbid depression and insomnia. Of the 43 patients in the study, 23 were randomized to the CBT-I group and 20 were randomized to the BAT-D group. With due consideration of the close functional relationship between insomnia and depression, the aim of this study was to evaluate the effect of CBT-I alone and BAT-D alone on both insomnia and depression and to evaluate the effects of each treatment on the other disorders. The results of the study demonstrated that CBT-I alone and BAT-D alone were efficacious for both insomnia and depression with, as might be expected, CBT-I being more efficacious for improving sleep and BAT-D being more efficacious in reducing depressive symptoms. Although this study did not fully isolate the effects of BAT-D on a pure insomnia sample, it shows how a BA protocol designed for depression can provide a level of treatment efficacy for insomnia.

WHAT THEORETIC FOUNDATION SUPPORTS THE USE OF BEHAVIORAL ACTIVATION IN INSOMNIA?

Although a complete analysis is beyond the scope of this article, a plausible rationale for BAs formal use in the treatment of insomnia can be constructed, nonetheless, informed by three rational elements:

Elements of Behavioral Activation Are Already Part of Standard Clinical Practice

Perhaps self-evident, BA is, at minimum, an incidental component in the standard practice of CBT-I. For example, patients undergoing CBT-I are commonly instructed to maintain the same 7-day-a-week time out of bed. This is often combined with the direction to start the day with exposure to robust circadian entrainers such as natural light, exercise, and taking of a morning meal. Arguably, these instructions are the effective components of insomnia treatment in themselves. However, a part of that effectiveness may be apportioned to the independent effects of BA that are in operation.

Insomnia and Depression May Share a Common Factor Responsive to Behavioral Activation

To the best of the author's knowledge, there are no factor analytical studies that have linked insomnia and depression to a common factor or factors. However, there are several places in the literature that provide evidence to support that insomnia and depression are, indeed, interrelated and places in the literature that suggest what factors may be operational in this linkage. For example, Sivertsen and colleagues,[19] in their analysis of 11 years of longitudinal data, found a robust bidirectional relationship between insomnia and depression. They determined that the presence of insomnia with no depression at baseline conferred a significant risk of depression developing over time and that the presence of depression with no insomnia at baseline conferred a significant risk of insomnia developing over time. Although this study demonstrates that insomnia and depression are clearly interrelated, it does not determine by what factors or mechanisms.

In speculating on potential factors and mechanisms that are instructive in this case, we may look to the work of Pigeon and Perlis[20] who proposed, for example, that the factor, *lack of control,* so common to the experience of insomnia, might play a role in the activation of depressive schemas such as helplessness and hopelessness. Similarly, Nagy and colleagues[21] argue that part of the effectiveness of BA may be attributable to its ability to target the factor, *anhedonia*—so common a symptom across many psychiatric disorders.

In this, we see the possibility that a BA protocol developed for depression might exert its effect on insomnia not only through the amelioration of the target, *depression* (if present), but also another common factor such as *anhedonia* or *lack of control*, as above, or another factor *superordinate* to anhedonia and lack of control that has yet to be determined.

Behavioral Activation Itself Is a Fundamental Mechanism of Change

In keeping with this thesis, DiMaggio and Shahar[22] argue that BA is not constrained to being simply a mode of treatment but elevated to a fundamental mechanism of change in psychotherapy, nearly parallel in standing to that of the therapeutic alliance. This reasoning comes from the finding that BA has shown efficacy across various disorders and types of psychotherapies indicating that BA clearly has utility beyond its original target of depression. This would then, of course, include support for its continued and perhaps, *expanded integration* into the treatment of insomnia.

FUNDAMENTAL CLINICAL CONCEPTS IN THE IMPLEMENTATION OF BEHAVIORAL ACTIVATION
Functional Analysis of Behavior

The functional analysis of behavior is a critical element in the deployment of BA. The purpose of a functional analysis is to identify the relationship between (1) *antecedents* to a behavior, (2) the *behavior* itself, and (3) the *consequences* of that behavior (see[23] for review). Effectively, all behavior can be examined using this system of inquiry, alternately referred to as Antecedent-Behavior-Consequence (ABC). To illustrate, let us consider a person who is observed drinking a glass of water. In this example, *thirst* is the antecedent, *drinking* is the behavior, and *stop drinking* is the observable consequence of a presumed state of satiety. Here, the ABC is Thirst- > Drinking- > Stop Drinking. In another situation, the antecedent might be different such that drinking a glass of water is not driven by thirst but by a dry mouth precipitated by anxiety leading to this ABC: Dry Mouth- > Drinking- > Stop Drinking. In each instance, this person is seen engaging in the same observable sequence but with different antecedents. It is understood that some events are private such as thoughts and internal sensations (thirst, dry mouth), and some are external and observable such as the behavior of drinking itself.

Core Clinical Principles of Behavioral Activation

BA draws on several core principles to support and guide the therapeutic process. Martell and colleagues[24] provide a comprehensive exposition of these core principles as they are to be applied in the treatment of depression. Selected elements of the principles outlined by Martell and colleagues are below and are adapted for the purposes of this article:

1. Act from the outside-in versus inside-out. The decision to engage in a valued behavior should not be guided by how one feels in the moment or whether one has sufficient motivation to act. Acting in this way is called acting from the *inside-out* because the decision to act is guided by an internal state or perception. Instead, one can make the decision to act guided by dedication to the valued behavior itself. Acting in this way is called acting from the *outside-in* because the outside valued behavior is given greater weight than a feeling at any given moment. A useful way to conceptualize is by noting that *behaviors should follow a plan, not a mood.*
2. Use a functional analysis of behaviors (the ABCs) to develop insight into the behavioral chain of events.
3. Begin with the smallest meaningful increment of behavioral change. Taking on too much increases the chance that a patient will fall short of a valued goal or, perhaps, not engage at all. Do not underestimate the reinforcing power of a small step in the right direction.
4. Approach the patient with compassion and punctuate that all results are useful. Much can be learned from failed attempts, and these should be met with understanding and empathy.

Behavioral Activation Is Not Just About "Getting Busy" or "Fixing Lazy Behavior"

With respect to both the theoretic underpinnings and clinical application of BA, it is important to distinguish BA from the oversimplified notion that just "getting busy" will be therapeutic. This "just get busy" exhortation may have been invoked many times over by concerned and well-meaning people trying to help. Despite good intentions, this kind of approach may, in the end, serve only to evoke a sense of guilt and shame in the patient for their apparent "failings," especially if attempts at behavior change have been unsuccessful. In a similar vein, it is also important to underscore that rushing aimlessly into the business of being busy for its own sake may be countertherapeutic if this busyness paves the road toward the avoidance of important feelings and behaviors.[24]

To help avoid these pitfalls, clinicians should make plain from the outset that the BA approach is not a remold of "getting busy," or "just do it," or that there is an assumption that the problem stems from laziness. Patients should be assured that great care will be given in developing behavioral targets that align with a patient's stated goals and values and that working in this way holds the potential to increase their sense of self-efficacy and agency.

APPLICATION OF BEHAVIORAL ACTIVATION TO THE TREATMENT OF INSOMNIA
Targets to Maintain a Consistent Wake Time

Sleeping past a prescribed wake time
A patient who is depressed or anxious will often endeavor to *sleep past* a prescribed wake time to delay waking into a full reemergence of distress. In addressing this, the clinician can help the patient appreciate that waking into this level of intense emotion is both common in this context and likely to pass as the morning routine unfolds. With that in mind, it can be useful to uncover some of the morning activities that might have been abandoned as the insomnia took hold and then evaluate which activities would be of the greatest therapeutic value to reinstate thereby reinforcing of a consistent wake time. Further, adding *additional* structure to the morning routine by including reliable exposure to circadian entrainers such as natural light, a morning meal, and some form of exercise should be considered.

Lingering in bed awake past a prescribed out of bed time
Lingering in bed *awake* past a prescribed wake time is another counterproductive behavior that can be addressed using BA. In the first few minutes post-wake, rising from bed can be particularly challenging.[3] The clinician can assist the patient by underscoring that this feeling is normal, whereas getting out of bed at a prescribed time

may come at a high emotional cost. It will ultimately give way to a lower cost, euthymic state. It is in this euthymic state that the patient can fully appreciate having accomplished something important and useful and this recognition lays the foundation for the positive reinforcement of the behavior.

Wake impeded by an exacerbation of sleep inertia

SC, SR, and the enforcement of a prescribed wake time are among the most potent behavioral elements of CBT-I. In combination, they serve to reduce conditioned arousal, entrain the circadian rhythm, and increase the homeostatic drive for sleep.[25,26] However, these benefits come with the short-term risk of increasing levels of sleepiness and sleep inertia at wake which can interfere with treatment compliance. In response to this, Kaplan and colleagues[27] developed a BA-based protocol to counterbalance this increase in sleep inertia, called RISE-UP. RISE-UP is an acronym that refers to the protocol's basic components, namely: (R) Refrain from snoozing, (I) Increase activity for the first hour, (S) Shower or wash face with cold water, (E) Exposure to sunlight, (U) Upbeat music, and (P) Phone a friend. This protocol was tested in a group of patients suffering from insomnia comorbid with bipolar disorder. In comparison to a habitual wake-up routine, the RISE-UP method was found to significantly reduce the duration and severity of self-reported sleep inertia, thereby supporting the treatment of insomnia.

Insomnia Comorbid with Depression: Special Considerations for the Use of Behavioral Activation

Behavioral activation to address the draw to an early bedtime in depression

Epidemiologic studies indicate that between 10% and 20% of persons diagnosed with insomnia also suffer from depression[28] and 80% of persons with a current major depressive episode present with insomnia symptoms. Patients struggling with insomnia comorbid with depression may be drawn toward an early bedtime as a strategy to escape from emotional pain. In addition to this avoidance being problematic in itself, the pull to escape to an early bedtime adds further difficulty to the proper deployment of SR especially when a substantially later time to bed is required. A way to address this would be to examine the kinds of evening activities that were typical before the insomnia began and then introduce them back into the nighttime routine.[3] The clinician may find it helpful to expand the nighttime behavioral

repertoire to include activities that assist the patient to remain awake until the prescribed time to bed.

Concurrent Treatment of Insomnia and Depression

BABIT as it is called is an integration of behavioral insomnia (SR and SC) and depression techniques (BA). This approach was developed to address the need to effectively treat depression comorbid with insomnia using a brief intervention model. Preliminary research indicates that BABIT has shown efficacy in reducing both depressive and insomnia symptoms.[29] Consider a patient who is prone to stay in bed resting instead of starting the day, a behavioral reaction common to both depression and insomnia. An initial approach here might be to discuss in detail how resting in bed contributes conditioned arousal and how rest cannot confer the benefits of sleep. This can then be followed by an explanation of how having a BA plan in place may provide sufficient incentive to exit the bed and bedroom and become active by engaging in zeitgebers such as a morning meal, exercise, and exposure to natural light. Although this is a difficult buy-in, a patient is likely to find that the protocol is reinforcing as activation in this way is both antidepressant and pro-sleep behaviors.

Out of Bed in the Middle of the Night: Behavioral Activation During Stimulus Control?

Standard instructions for SC are often as follows: Engage in a quiet activity under low light. This is generally a reasonable place to start and is very much in line with the fundamental spirit of SC. However, when patients complain that being up and out of bed in the middle of the night is just miserable, other notions about what behaviors and activities are advisable should be explored. Although engaging in activities that create needless agitation should always be discouraged, activities that foster a sense of present moment contentment should not, even if those activities are arguably energizing or entertaining. For example, the middle of the night might be good time to watch a favorite movie or catch up on some amusing reading. The patient who begins to understand that being up in the middle of the night is not inextricably tied to frustration, and misery is a patient who will begin to develop less agitation around the prospect of waking in the first place and more likely to relax in a way that unmasks sleepiness.

Behavioral Activation: Daytime Function and Overall Quality of Life

Most people with insomnia experience some level of mental and physical fatigue and, in response, place unneeded limits on their level of activity. For some, this is a response to a perceived need to conserve energy, and for some, this is simply a response to diminished motivation. Often this simply comes down to: "I can't do it" or "I don't feel like doing it." Expanding our descriptors beyond fatigue, Kyle and colleagues[30] set to explore the phenomenology of people with chronically disturbed sleep. In their study, qualitative data from focus groups and audio diaries were analyzed and the following categories emerged as among the self-descriptors identified: "just struggle through," "isolated, feeling like an outsider," and "insomnia as an obstruction to the desired self." These are sober findings, powerful and telling descriptions that match well with what is heard in clinic routinely. BA can be a valuable adjunct toward helping address these specific issues.

In evaluating targets for treatment, a useful question to ask patients is: "what would you be doing if you felt better?" The answers can help the patient reconsider how their behavioral repertoire has changed in response to their insomnia and how that has affected quality of life. The clinician can start by having the patient consider the behaviors that have come to mind and apply the ABCs (core principle 2). For example, a patient may routinely cancel plans (Behavior) with friends when fatigued (Antecedent) leading to a temporary relief of stress (Consequence)—maintained by negative reinforcement. The patient also recognizes how canceling plans has led to demoralization and is motivated to find a way to reverse the pattern. Here, the decision to be with friends should be guided by the plan in place and not a mood (core principle 1). In choosing a plan, the clinician can work with the patient to find the smallest meaningful increment of change (core principle 3) —say, having coffee with a friend just 1 day during the week. If the patient falls short of this goal, remind the patient that all results are useful (core principle 4) and begin an exploration of what factors may have hindered the plan.

Integration of Social Rhythms and Behavioral Activation

The application of BA to insomnia is made more complete by a full consideration of how the rhythmicity of activity and not just activity itself contributes to sleep health. The regularization of social rhythms has been found to be significant factor in improving sleep.[31–33] Sabet and colleagues[34] determined that overall sleep health as defined by Buysse[35] is linked to both mental health and social rhythm regularity. Specifically, they found that the regularity of social rhythms is directly associated with fewer symptoms of anxiety and depression and that this relationship is mediated by healthy sleep behaviors and thoughts. Research on social rhythms punctuate the notion that both the timing and rhythmicity of activities, not just the activities themselves, are central in themselves and are central to maximizing the benefits of BA.

Closing Remarks

Sustained commitment to valued and pleasurable activities despite fatigue and low mood can promote a healthy adaptation to poor sleep and is among the primary positive effects associated with using BA as an adjunct to standard insomnia treatment. A patient who develops a measure of agency in their relationship to both daytime and nighttime experience is a patient who may now experience a lessening of the need to excessively focus on sleep because sleep is now seen as only one of several factors contributing to mental and physical function—"I know it's now possible to have a good day and a good night even if my sleep is poor." Less focus on sleep in this way can also reduce counterproductive self-monitoring, sleep effort, and other sources of nighttime distress, reducing arousal, and promoting sleep.

Developing a more complete understanding of the independent contribution that BA confers to the treatment of insomnia would allow its more informed usage. This level of refinement of our understanding of BA in the context of insomnia will help to optimize our implementation into clinical practice much in the same way that our expanded understanding of the independent effects of SR and SC has benefitted treatment.

CLINICS CARE POINTS

- Behavioral activation (BA) can be used to support CBT-I by improving adherence to pleasurable and personally valuable activities which can improve daytime function and mood.

- Increases in activity and greater rhythmicity/regularity of activity may increase homeostatic sleep drive and enhance circadian entrainment.

- BA can be applied to help promote adherence to prescribed rise and wake times and compliance with a later time to bed prescribed in the course of sleep restriction.
- Behavioral Activation and Behavioral Insomnia Therapy for insomnia comorbid with depression and RISE-UP for sleep inertia are useful treatments to consider that formally integrate BA into the treatment of insomnia.

DISCLOSURE

No conflicts of interest to disclose.

REFERENCES

1. Perlis ML. Cognitive behavioral treatment of insomnia : a session-by-session guide/Michael L. Perlis [and others]. New York, NY: Springer; 2005.
2. Perlis ML, Aloia M, Kuhn BR. Behavioral treatments for sleep disorders a comprehensive primer of behavioral sleep medicine interventions/. In: Michael P, Mark A, Brett K, editors. Practical resources for the mental health professional. 1st edition. Elsevier; 2011. p. 2–3.
3. Manber R, Carney CE. Treatment plans and interventions for insomnia : a case formulation approach/Rachel Manber, *Colleen E. Carney*. Treatment plans and interventions for evidence-based psychotherapy. New York, NY: The Guilford Press; 2015.
4. Bootzin RR. Stimulus control treatment for insomnia. Proc Am Psychol Assoc 1972;7:395–6.
5. Spielman AJ, Saskin P, Thorpy MJ. Treatment of chronic insomnia by restriction of time in bed. Sleep 1987;10(1):45–56.
6. Hayes SC. A liberated mind: how to pivot toward what matters. London, UK: Penguin Publishing Group; 2019.
7. Ferster CB. A functional analysis of depression. Am Psychol 1973;28(10):857–70.
8. Lewinsohn PM, Libet J. Pleasant events, activity schedules, and depressions. J Abnorm Psychol 1972;79(3):291–5.
9. Ciharova M, Furukawa TA, Efthimiou O, et al. Cognitive restructuring, behavioral activation and cognitive-behavioral therapy in the treatment of adult depression: a network meta-analysis. J Consul Clin Psychol 2021;89(6):563–74.
10. Cuijpers P, van Straten A, Warmerdam L. Behavioral activation treatments of depression: a meta-analysis. Clin Psychol Rev 2007;27(3):318–26.
11. Dimidjian S, Hollon SD, Dobson KS, et al. Randomized trial of behavioral activation, cognitive therapy, and antidepressant medication in the acute treatment of adults with major depression. J Consult Clin Psychol 2006;74(4):658–70.
12. Farchione TJ, Boswell JF, Wilner JG. Behavioral activation strategies for major depression in transdiagnostic cognitive-behavioral therapy: an evidence-based case study. Psychotherapy 2017; 54(3):225–30.
13. Sturmey P. Behavioral activation is an evidence-based treatment for depression. Behav Modif 2009;33(6):818–29.
14. Jacobson NS, Dobson KS, Truax PA, et al. A component analysis of cognitive-behavioral treatment for depression. J Consul Clin Psychol 1996; 64(2):295–304.
15. Diagnostic and statistical manual of mental disorders : DSM-5. 5th edition. ed. DSM-5. Washington (DC): American Psychiatric Association; 2013.
16. Sateia M. International classification of sleep disorders/American academy of sleep medicine. 3rd edition. Darien, IL: ICSD. American Academy of Sleep Medicine; 2014.
17. Yi XX. Behavioral Activation for improving sleep quality in family caregivers of people with dementia: a pilot randomized controlled trial. Dissertation. Hung Hom, Hong Kong: The Hong Kong Polytechnic University; 2020.
18. Lin C, Lane H, Huang C, et al. A comparison of treatment outcome of cognitive behavioral therapy for insomnia (CBT-I) and behavioral activation therapy for depression (BAT-D) in patients with comorbid depression and insomnia. Sleep Med 2015;16:S259.
19. Sivertsen B, Salo P, Mykletun A, et al. The bidirectional association between depression and insomnia: the HUNT study. Psychosom Med 2012;74(7):758–65.
20. Pigeon WR, Perlis ML. Insomnia and depression: birds of a feather? Journal. Int J Sleep Disord 2007;1:82–91.
21. Nagy GA, Cernasov P, Pisoni A, et al. Reward network modulation as a mechanism of change in behavioral activation. Behav Modif 2020;44(2): 186–213.
22. Dimaggio G, Shahar G. Behavioral activation as a common mechanism of change across different orientations and disorders. Psychotherapy (Chic) 2017;54(3):221–4.
23. Rozycki EG. The functional analysis of behavior. Educ Theory 1975;25(3):278–302.
24. Martell C, Dimidjian S, Herman-Dunn R. Behavioral activation for depression. New York, NY: The Guilford Press; 2022.
25. Cervena K, Dauvilliers Y, Espa F, et al. Effect of cognitive behavioural therapy for insomnia on sleep architecture and sleep EEG power spectra in psychophysiological insomnia. J Sleep Res 2004; 13(4):385–93.
26. Pigeon WR, Perlis ML. Sleep homeostasis in primary insomnia. Sleep Med Rev 2006;10(4):247–54.

27. Kaplan KA, Talavera DC, Harvey AG. Rise and shine: a treatment experiment testing a morning routine to decrease subjective sleep inertia in insomnia and bipolar disorder. Behav Res Ther 2018;111:106–12.

28. Ohayon MM. Insomnia: a ticking clock for depression? J Psychiatr Res 2007;41(11):893–4.

29. Carney CE, Posner D. Cognitive behavior therapy for insomnia in those with depression: a guide for clinicians. New York, NY: Routledge; 2015.

30. Kyle SD, Espie CA, Morgan K. Not just a minor thing, it is something major, which stops you from functioning daily": quality of life and daytime functioning in insomnia. Behav Sleep Med 2010;8(3):123–40.

31. Moss TG, Carney CE, Haynes P, et al. Is daily routine important for sleep? An investigation of social rhythms in a clinical insomnia population. Chronobiol Int 2015;32(1):92–102.

32. Carney CE, Edinger JD, Meyer B, et al. Daily activities and sleep quality in college students. Chronobiol Int 2006;23(3):623–37.

33. Haynes PL, Kelly M, Warner L, et al. Cognitive Behavioral Social Rhythm Group Therapy for Veterans with posttraumatic stress disorder, depression, and sleep disturbance: results from an open trial. J affective Disord 2015;192:234–43.

34. Sabet SM, Dautovich ND, Dzierzewski JM. The rhythm is gonna get you: social rhythms, sleep, depressive, and anxiety symptoms. J affective Disord 2021;286:197–203.

35. Buysse DJ. Sleep health: can we define it? Does it matter? Sleep (New York, NY) 2014;37(1):9–17.

Exercise as an Adjunct Treatment to Cognitive Behavior Therapy for Insomnia

Giselle Soares Passos, PhD[a],*, Shawn D. Youngstedt, PhD[b],
Marcos Gonçalves Santana, PhD[a]

KEYWORDS

• Physical activity • Insomnia • Sleep • Non-drug therapy

KEY POINTS

• Cognitive behavioral therapy for insomnia (CBT-I) is the first-line treatment of insomnia, but it does not work for as many as 30% to 40% of patients.
• Exercise has been recommended as an adjuvant therapy for chronic insomnia.
• Improvements on sleep, mood and insomnia severity are reported with moderate- to vigorous-intensity aerobic exercise, moderate-intensity resistance exercise and stretching, for at least 150 min/wk.
• Clinical trials assessing exercise added to CBT-I for chronic insomnia are needed.

INTRODUCTION

Epidemiologic studies have shown about one-third of the general population have at least one symptom of chronic insomnia and 7% to 10% are diagnosed with insomnia disorder, based on diagnostic and statistical manual of mental disorders (DSM) and international classification of sleep disorders (ICSD) criteria.[1,2] Insomnia has been associated with mortality[3] and much morbidity, including coronary heart disease,[4] hypertension,[5] heart failure,[6] depression, and anxiety.[7]

Cognitive behavior therapy for insomnia (CBT-I) is the first-line treatment of chronic insomnia. Traditionally, CBT-I has been applied *in person* (individual or in group) by a trained psychologist/clinician, in about four-eight sessions, that usually focus on sleep restriction therapy, stimulus-control principles, sleep hygiene education, relaxation, and cognitive therapy.[8] Multiple reviews and comparative efficacy trials have shown that CBT-I is superior to hypnotics for chronic treatment of insomnia.[9,10] Moreover, recent research has shown similar effects when administered remotely and even online (self-help/Internet based).[9] Brief behavioral treatment for chronic insomnia (BBT-I) has also been effective when applied in the primary care setting, even by providers who are not sleep medicine specialists.[11,12]

However, some key barriers have been reported for CBT-I, including effectiveness, knowledge, beliefs, access, adherence, therapeutic failure, and access to providers.[13] Side-effects of CBT-I, including increases in somnolence, fatigue and objectively impaired vigilance due to the sleep restriction component of CBT-I[9] are also barriers to treatment. Indeed, some studies indicate that for a significant percent of patients CBT-I is not effective. For example, Morin and colleagues[14] found no response in 40% of patients and absence of remission in 58% of patients who received CBT-I for 6 weeks. Likewise, Koffel and colleagues[13] reported that 20% to 30% of patients treated with CBT-I did not experience significant improvements in sleep. Another study found that 19% to 26% of participants failed to show any response to treatment with CBT-I.[15]

[a] Health Sciences Unit, Universidade Federal de Jataí, BR 364, km 195, n. 3800, CEP 75801-61, Jataí- GO, Brazil;
[b] Edson College of Nursing and Health Innovation, Arizona State University, 550 N 3rd Road Street, Phoenix, AZ 85004, USA
* Corresponding author.
E-mail address: passos.gs@gmail.com

Sleep Med Clin 18 (2023) 39–47
https://doi.org/10.1016/j.jsmc.2022.09.001
1556-407X/23/© 2022 Elsevier Inc. All rights reserved.

Moreover, some evidence indicates that individuals with insomnia who sleep ≤ 6 h are less likely to be responsive to CBT-I than those sleeping more than 6 h,[16,17] which might be explained by difficulty (and risk) that the sleep restriction component (see below) of CBT-I might have for short sleepers.

Thus, adjuvant treatments would be helpful. In the present paper, we review the evidence that exercise improves chronic insomnia, and we discuss rationales for combining CBT-I with exercise.

EVIDENCE THAT EXERCISE CAN BE A TREATMENT OF CHRONIC INSOMNIA

Since the 1990s, the effects of exercise on insomnia have been investigated.[18–25] The first review articles suggesting insomnia as the best model to study the effects of exercise on sleep were published in the 2000s,[26,27] but only after 10 years were the first clinical trials published.[23,25] Chronic[18,20–22,25] and acute[23,28] exercise have elicited improvements or no impairment[19] on sleep in patients with chronic insomnia. Systematic reviews report improvements on sleep in patients with insomnia disorder,[29–33] insomnia symptoms,[29] and chronic insomnia related to menopause.[34] Exercise has been recommended as adjunct therapy in the European Guideline for the Diagnosis and Treatment of Insomnia.[9]

Acute Effects

Acute effects (single night) of exercise and sleep have been investigated. The effects of three modalities of exercise (moderate-intensity aerobic exercise 'walking on a treadmill', high-intensity aerobic exercise 'running on a treadmill', and moderate-intensity resistance exercise) on sleep were examined in adult patients with chronic primary insomnia. The polysomnographic data showed significant reduction in sleep onset latency (SOL) and total wake time; and an increase in total sleep time (TST) and sleep efficiency (SE), after moderate-intensity aerobic exercise. The daily sleep log data showed an increase in self-reported TST and a reduction in SOL. In addition, decreases in the pre-sleep anxiety states were observed after the moderate intensity aerobic exercise.[23]

The effects of morning versus evening exercise (aerobic step exercise) on sleep in older individuals with insomnia was examined. No significant improvements were observed in sleep quality. The authors reported morning exercise decreased the number of stage shifts over the whole night. The arousal index and the number of stage shifts were decreased especially during the second half of the night in all groups. Morning exercise decreased the number of wake stages during the second half of the night in patients with difficulty in initiating sleep.[28]

The effects of nighttime exercise were studied in patients with insomnia compared with a control quiet reading treatment. The protocol included 30 min of moderate treadmill exercise plus 15 min of moderate resistance exercise, 2 h before bedtime. No significant treatment differences in sleep were found; however, two participants had severely disturbed objective sleep following exercise. Significant correlations were found between change in state anxiety from pre-exercise to bedtime and TST, Stage 1, wake time after sleep onset (WASO), and SE. Data provides some support for caution regarding late-night exercise for sedentary individuals with insomnia.[19]

The Effects of Chronic Exercise

The efficacy of 16 weeks of moderate aerobic exercise (walking, stationary bicycle, or treadmill), 30 to 40 min, four times per week, on sleep in older adults with chronic insomnia was assessed. The authors reported improvements in sleep quality, SOL, sleep duration, daytime dysfunction and sleep efficiency pittsburgh sleep quality index (PSQI) sub-scores, compared with a control treatment. In addition, reductions in depressive symptoms, daytime sleepiness, and improvements in vitality after exercise training compared with baseline were reported.[25]

The effects of 6 months morning versus late-afternoon moderate intensity aerobic exercise (walking on a treadmill), for 50 min on sleep, mood and quality of life in patients with chronic primary insomnia was assessed. A significant decrease in SOL and WASO and a significant increase in SE were observed following exercise training. Data from sleep diaries revealed significant improvement in SOL, sleep quality and feeling rested in the morning. Following exercise, some quality-of-life measures improved significantly, and a significant decrease was observed on tension-anxiety, depression and total mood disturbance. There were generally no significant differences in response between morning and late-afternoon exercise.[22]

Alterations on markers of immune function and hyperarousal were observed after moderate-intensity aerobic exercise (walking on a treadmill), for 50 min, for 4 months. In addition to sleep improvements, data showed significant increase in plasma apolipoprotein A, decreases in CD4, CD8, and plasma cortisol. Significant correlation was observed between decreases in cortisol and increases in total sleep time and REM sleep.[20]

Moderate intensity resistance exercise (focusing on the upper and lower limbs, abdominals, and paravertebral areas) for 4 months was assessed in patients with chronic insomnia. No significant treatment differences between resistance exercise and stretching, three times a week were observed. However, compared with the control (non-intervention), resistance exercise and stretching led to significantly greater improvements in insomnia severity, actigraphic measures of SOL, WASO and SE and sleep quality.[21]

Some additional evidence indicates that increasing the physical activity level (to $\geq$ 150 min of moderate-to-vigorous-intensity physical activity per week) improves sleep and mood[18] and psychomotor performance in people with insomnia.[35] Other interventions focused on increase of the physical activity level have been studied to reduce insomnia symptoms, like Zero-time exercise.[36] It is a lifestyle integrated exercise created to promote the incorporation of simple exercises into daily life and habituated activities. For example,: corporal movements are performed to simulate traditional exercise, such as 'cycling in the air'.

RATIONALES FOR COMBINING COGNITIVE BEHAVIOR THERAPY FOR INSOMNIA WITH EXERCISE

Acute daytime exercise and chronic exercise are almost invariably included in sleep hygiene education, which also includes recommendations such as avoiding caffeine (particularly afternoon), tobacco and alcohol use; managing stress and noise, avoiding daytime napping, having a regular sleep schedule; and performing quiet activities before bedtime. However, sleep hygiene education is the least emphasized component of CBT-I. Indeed, in measures of adherence to CBT-I, the focus has been almost entirely on sleep restriction and keeping a stable wake time (see below). Nonetheless, there are rationales for further emphasizing exercise for reasons discussed above. Exercise could also facilitate the following other components of CBT-I.

Sleep Restriction and Homeostatic Sleep Drive

Sleep restriction therapy (SRT) is thought to be perhaps the most crucial component of CBT-I.[37] There is variability in the SRT method, but in general it consists of a systematic reduction of time-in-bed (TIB, sleep window) of patients to the amount self-reported total sleep duration plus an average of 30 min - to account for wakefulness (SOL and WASO)[37–39] that occurs during the time in bed.

One key mechanism by which sleep restriction is believed to promote sleep is by promoting the homeostatic sleep drive,[40] which is evidenced by increases in sleep duration and deep sleep. Homeostatic sleep drive or pressure for sleep builds up as time awake increases. The pressure gets stronger the longer one stays awake and decreases during sleep, reaching a low after a full night of good-quality sleep. The homeostatic process begins to build again after we awaken.

One drawback regarding sleep restriction is that it can elicit sleepiness and fatigue. The majority of studies did not specify the minimum sleep window time, but the most frequent procedures are based on a 5 h minimum TIB, though some studies have reported a minimum of 4 h TIB.[37]

There is some evidence that exercise might be an effective adjunct for sleep restriction. Exercise could be particularly helpful for individuals with insomnia and short sleep duration (<6 h) that shown a poor response to CBT-I. Exercise increases sleep pressure, as evidenced by increased sleep duration (on the subsequent night-acute effect[22] and sustained for long-term exercise training[20,25]) and deep sleep (reported previously for good sleepers after acute and chronic exercise[26,41]). In addition, both moderate acute and chronic exercise elicit decreases in fatigue.[42,43] Adding exercise to CBT-I can be an alternative to minimize the poor adherence of patients with short sleep duration to CBT-I.

Sleep restriction and circadian synchronization

There is increasing evidence that having an erratic sleep/wake schedule is associated with poor sleep, and a trend for delayed sleep and social jet lag. One key feature of SRT is that it requires the patient to get up at the same time each day. The rationale for this requirement is that it helps promote circadian synchronization.[40] Exercise can shift rhythms and help stabilize the circadian system. Youngstedt and colleagues[44] reported that both morning and afternoon exercise can advance the body clock, which could be helpful in the treatment of sleep onset insomnia.

Conditioning

Another concept of CBT-I, particularly of stimulus-control training, is strengthening the association of the bed and bedroom environment with sleep. Instructions include i) go to bed only when sleepy; ii) use the bed only for sleeping and sexual activity (no reading, TV, eating, or working in bed); iii) if unable to fall asleep, either at the beginning or in the middle of the night, get out of bed and return to bed only when sleepy again. iv) avoid excessive napping during the day. This training is based on the premise that insomnia is a conditioned response to temporal (time spent in bed) and environmental (bedroom/bed) factors related to sleep. Its main objective is to strengthen the association of the bedroom and falling asleep faster and staying asleep. Therefore, activities incompatible with sleep should be abbreviated (observable and camouflaged, used as cues to stay awake).

Exercise could promote conditioning by providing a greater contrast of activity during sleep and wake. Exercise in the morning or evening could help avoid spending time in bed but not sleeping.

Hyperarousal and Insomnia

Hyperarousal during sleep and wakefulness is thought to be a significant etiologic and perpetuating factor for chronic insomnia.[45,46] This theory includes both physiologic (eg, elevated heart rate) and cognitive arousal (eg, an 'overactive' mind), which compromise the ability to fall asleep.[45] CBT-I aims to reduce hyperarousal via strategies such as relaxation therapy, SRT and Stimulus control.[47] However, physiologic hyperarousal cannot respond strongly or durably to CBT-I.[48] In accordance, a recent review provided less robust evidence in support of hyperarousal as a mediator of effects of CBT-I on chronic insomnia.[47] In addition, a previous study has observed no effects on delta, sigma and beta power during NREM sleep at post-treatment with CBT-I.[49] Exercise is effective in reducing psychophysiological arousal[19,26,50,51] and added to CBT-I could improve its effects.

Health

It has been speculated that CBT-I can improve health, and studies show some promising support for this hypothesis. Reductions in inflammation[52,53] and improvements in glucose regulation[54] and reported health[55] have been found following CBT-I. In addition, CBT-I reduces depression[48] and anxiety,[56] and improves physical and mental functioning and quality of life of patients with chronic insomnia.[13,57] Although there is potential risk of CBT-I associated with increased daytime sleepiness,[54] CBT-I is an effective and durable non-drug therapy that may increase the effectiveness of positive airway pressure (PAP) therapy.[58]

However, clearly exercise has overwhelming health benefits which would likely further promote these effects. Moderate-intensity aerobic exercise improves immune function[20,59] in patients with chronic insomnia. Some clinical trials have also reported significant reduction in depression symptoms following regular moderate-intensity aerobic exercise[18,20,22,25] in patients with chronic insomnia. In addition, decreases in anxiety symptoms have also been observed following regular moderate-intensity aerobic exercise,[18,22] and pre-sleep anxiety reductions are reported after an acute session of moderate-intensity aerobic exercise.[23] Reduction in anxiety has been observed also after a 4-month stretching program.[21] In patients enrolled in a cardiac rehabilitation, greater insomnia severity predicted greater improvements during exercise in both overall mood state and tranquility, following statistical adjustment for demographic variables and pre-exercise mood state.[60] A recent survey reported that good sleep health and high levels of physical activity were both individually associated with fewer depression symptoms. Sleep health significantly mediated 19% of the association between physical activity and depression symptoms, whereas physical activity significantly mediated 3% of the relationship between sleep health and depression symptoms.[61]

Obstructive sleep apnea (OSA) can co-occur with insomnia in some patients.[62] The effects of exercise on OSA are well established in the literature.[63] A meta-analysis identified a significant effect of exercise in reducing the apnea-hypopnea index (AHI) in patients with OSA, despite the minimal change in body mass. Furthermore, significant effects of physical exercise on cardiovascular fitness, daytime sleepiness and SE were observed, indicating the potential value of physical exercise in the treatment of OSA.[63] Kline and colleagues[64] reported a significant reduction in AHI and oxygen saturation, as well as an increase in N3 after 12 weeks of intervention with aerobic exercise associated with resistance exercise, in overweight/obese patients with moderate OSA (AHI>15), untreated. Weight loss is clearly a mechanism by which physical exercise can help prevent and treat OSA, although several studies indicate an inverse relationship between exercise practice and OSA severity, regardless of the body mass index. Another hypothesis suggested is that during exercise there may be strengthening of the oropharyngeal muscles, making them less susceptible to collapse associated with upper airway obstruction during sleep.[26]

HOW COGNITIVE BEHAVIOR THERAPY FOR INSOMNIA COULD ADD TO THE EFFECTS OF EXERCISE ON INSOMNIA

Notwithstanding the benefits of acute and chronic exercise for insomnia, to our knowledge, exercise is not prescribed as a stand-alone treatment of insomnia. As discussed above, many features of

Table 1
Exercise treatment protocols

	Type	Frequency	Intensity	Duration	Time of Day
Reid et al,[25] 2010	aerobic exercise: walking, stationary bicycle, or treadmill.	Four times/wk	75% HRmax	30–40 min	1–7 PM
Passos et al,[23] 2010	aerobic exercise: walking on a treadmill	One session	VT1	50 min	6 PM
Passos et al,[22] 2011	aerobic exercise: walking on a treadmill	Three times/wk	VT1	50 min	10 ± 1 AM or 6 ± 1 PM
Morita et al,[28] 2017	aerobic step exercise with 5-min rest periods between sets.	One session	Moderate	Four sets of 10 min	9:30 AM to 11 AM or 5:30 PM 7 PM
Hartescu et al,[18] 2015	brisk walking	Five times/wk	Moderate	At least 30 min	n/a
D'Aurea et al,[21] 2019	resistance exercise: each session included four exercises for the upper limbs (biceps, triceps, back, and pectorals); four exercises for the lower limbs (flexors, extensors, abductors, and adductors); one trunk flexion exercise for the abdominal area; and one trunk extension exercise for the paravertebral area (spinal stabilizers). Each exercise was performed in three series of 12 repetitions with 30-s intervals between series and 1-min intervals between the different types of exercise.	Three times/wk	50%–60% 1RM	50 min	5 PM
D'Aurea et al,[21] 2019	Stretching: each session included 5-min walk around the room, followed by 45 min of stretching exercises involving the upper and lower limbs, with 8–10 types for each body region.	Three imes/wk	n/a	50 min	5 PM

Notes: HRmax (maximum heart rate), VT1 (ventilatory Threshold 1),[66,67] n/a (not applicable).

CBT-I could potentiate effects of exercise on insomnia. The goal of cognitive therapy into CBT-I is to eliminate beliefs and wrong attitudes related to sleep[65] including (i) a false concept of adequate sleep time ("I can't sleep 8 h that are necessary for my well-being..."); (ii) an inadequate conception of the causes of insomnia ("My insomnia is a chemistry consequence..."); (iii) Amplification of insomnia consequences ("I can do nothing after a bad night's sleep..."). Cognitive therapy is also used to reduce cognitive arousal by helping patients shift from "trying hard to sleep" to "allowing sleep to happen." As exercise is not likely to work well for some of the factors that contribute to insomnia such as beliefs and wrong attitudes related to sleep, combining these therapies can result in more effective improvements on insomnia.

SUMMARY

Considering the similar improvements mediated by CBT-I alone and exercise alone on insomnia, we were motivated to write the ways to consider adding exercise to CBT-I. Exercise has been recommended as adjuvant therapy, although the evidence has been judged to be of low quality.[8] The improvements observed in clinical trials in the last 10 years show that exercise can be an effective adjuvant treatment of chronic insomnia. Regular exercise is a recommendation included in sleep hygiene education, and sleep hygiene education is a component of CBT-I. In this way, exercise is a sub-component of CBT-I. Giving more attention to exercise prescription could result in more benefits for the health of patients. The exercise recommendation should be based in the published studies showing improvements on sleep/insomnia of patients (**Table 1**). Exercise added to CBT-I can improve its effects on sleep drive, circadian synchronization, conditioning, and health. On the other hand, especially the cognitive components of CBT-I could add to the effects of exercise on insomnia.

CLINICS CARE POINTS

- Cognitive behavioral therapy for insomnia (CBT-I) is the first-line treatment of chronic insomnia. Adjunct alternative treatments to CBT-I could be welcome, in case of no access, no adherence or therapeutic failure.

- Although considering exercise is included in sleep hygiene education and this is a frequent component of CBT-I, more attention to exercise prescription could be relevant.

- Despite limited evidence, exercise has shown significant improvement on sleep of patients with insomnia disorder.

- No treatment is perfect for insomnia. CBT-I has limitations. Exercise is not likely to work as well for some of the factors that contribute to insomnia, such as beliefs, etc. There are good rationales for combining CBT-I with exercise.

DISCLOSURE

All authors declare no commercial or financial conflicts of interest and any funding source.

REFERENCES

1. Ohayon MM, Reynolds CF 3rd. Epidemiological and clinical relevance of insomnia diagnosis algorithms according to the DSM-IV and the International Classification of Sleep Disorders (ICSD). Sleep Med 2009;10(9):952–60.
2. National Institutes of H. National Institutes of health state of the science Conference statement on Manifestations and Management of chronic insomnia in adults, June 13-15, 2005. Sleep 2005;28(9):1049–57.
3. Lovato N, Lack L. Insomnia and mortality: a meta-analysis. Sleep Med Rev 2019;43:71–83.
4. Javaheri S, Redline S. Insomnia and risk of cardiovascular disease. Chest 2017;152(2):435–44.
5. Jarrin DC, Alvaro PK, Bouchard MA, et al. Insomnia and hypertension: a systematic review. Sleep Med Rev 2018;41:3–38.
6. Laugsand LE, Strand LB, Platou C, et al. Insomnia and the risk of incident heart failure: a population study. Eur Heart J 2014;35(21):1382–93.
7. Neckelmann D, Mykletun A, Dahl AA. Chronic insomnia as a risk factor for developing anxiety and depression. Sleep 2007;30(7):873–80.
8. Riemann D, Perlis ML. The treatments of chronic insomnia: a review of benzodiazepine receptor agonists and psychological and behavioral therapies. Sleep Med Rev 2009;13(3):205–14.
9. Riemann D, Baglioni C, Bassetti C, et al. European guideline for the diagnosis and treatment of insomnia. J Sleep Res 2017;26(6):675–700.
10. Qaseem A, Kansagara D, Forciea MA, Cooke M, Denberg TD. Clinical Guidelines Committee of the American College of P. Management of Chronic Insomnia Disorder in Adults: A Clinical Practice Guideline From the American College of Physicians. Annals of Internal Medicine 2016;165(2):125–33. https://doi.org/10.7326/M15-2175.
11. Gunn HE, Tutek J, Buysse DJ. Brief Behavioral Treatment of Insomnia. Sleep Medicine Clinics 2019;

14(2):235–43. https://doi.org/10.1016/j.jsmc.2019.
02.003.

12. Buysse DJ, Germain A, Moul DE, et al. Efficacy of brief
behavioral treatment for chronic insomnia in older
adults. Archives of Internal Medicine 2011;171(10):
887–95. https://doi.org/10.1001/archinternmed.
2010.535.

13. Koffel E, Bramoweth AD, Ulmer CS. Increasing access to and utilization of cognitive behavioral therapy for insomnia (CBT-I): a narrative review.
Journal of General Internal Medicine 2018;33(6):
955–62. https://doi.org/10.1007/s11606-018-4390-1.

14. Morin CM, Vallieres A, Guay B, et al. Cognitive
behavioral therapy, singly and combined with medication, for persistent insomnia: a randomized
controlled trial. JAMA 2009;301(19):2005–15.
https://doi.org/10.1001/jama.2009.682.

15. Harvey AG, Tang NK. Cognitive behaviour therapy
for primary insomnia: can we rest yet? Sleep Medicine Reviews 2003;7(3):237–62. https://doi.org/10.
1053/smrv.2002.0266.

16. Bastien CH, Ellis JG, Grandner M. CBT-I and the
short sleep duration insomnia phenotype: a
comment on Bathgate, Edinger and Krystal. Annals
of Translational Medicine 2017;5(16):335. https://doi.
org/10.21037/atm.2017.04.27.

17. Bathgate CJ, Edinger JD, Krystal AD. Insomnia Patients With Objective Short Sleep Duration Have a
Blunted Response to Cognitive Behavioral Therapy
for Insomnia. Sleep 2017;40(1). https://doi.org/10.
1093/sleep/zsw012.

18. Hartescu I, Morgan K, Stevinson CD. Increased
physical activity improves sleep and mood outcomes
in inactive people with insomnia: a randomized
controlled trial. Journal of Sleep Research 2015;
24(5):526–34. https://doi.org/10.1111/jsr.12297.

19. Youngstedt SD, Ito W, Passos GS, Santana MG,
Youngstedt JM. Testing the sleep hygiene recommendation against nighttime exercise. Sleep &
Breathing = Schlaf & Atmung 2021. https://doi.org/
10.1007/s11325-020-02284-x.

20. Passos GS, Poyares D, Santana MG, et al. Exercise
improves immune function, antidepressive
response, and sleep quality in patients with chronic
primary insomnia. BioMed Research International
2014;2014:498961. https://doi.org/10.1155/2014/
498961.

21. D'Aurea CVR, Poyares D, Passos GS, et al. Effects
of resistance exercise training and stretching on
chronic insomnia. Braz J Psychiatry 2019;41(1):
51–7. https://doi.org/10.1590/1516-4446-2018-0030.

22. Passos GS, Poyares D, Santana MG, et al. Effects of
moderate aerobic exercise training on chronic primary insomnia. Sleep Medicine 2011;12(10):
1018–27. https://doi.org/10.1016/j.sleep.2011.02.007.

23. Passos GS, Poyares D, Santana MG, Garbuio SA,
Tufik S, Mello MT. Effect of acute physical exercise

on patients with chronic primary insomnia. Journal
of Clinical Sleep Medicine 2010;6(3):270–5.

24. Baron KG, Reid KJ, Zee PC. Exercise to improve
sleep in insomnia: exploration of the bidirectional effects. Journal of clinical Sleep Medicine 2013;9(8):
819–24. https://doi.org/10.5664/jcsm.2930.

25. Reid KJ, Baron KG, Lu B, Naylor E, Wolfe L, Zee PC.
Aerobic exercise improves self-reported sleep and
quality of life in older adults with insomnia. Sleep
Medicine 2010;11(9):934–40. https://doi.org/10.
1016/j.sleep.2010.04.014.

26. Youngstedt SD. Effects of exercise on sleep. Clin
Sports Med 2005;24(2):355–65, xi.

27. Driver HS, Taylor SR. Exercise and sleep. Sleep
Medicine Reviews 2000;4(4):387–402.

28. Morita Y, Sasai-Sakuma T, Inoue Y. Effects of acute
morning and evening exercise on subjective and
objective sleep quality in older individuals with
insomnia. Sleep Medicine 2017;34:200–8. https://
doi.org/10.1016/j.sleep.2017.03.014.

29. Lowe H, Haddock G, Mulligan LD, et al. Does exercise improve sleep for adults with insomnia? A systematic review with quality appraisal. Clinical
Psychology Review 2019;68:1–12. https://doi.org/
10.1016/j.cpr.2018.11.002.

30. Li S, Li Z, Wu Q, et al. Effect of exercise intervention
on primary insomnia: a meta-analysis. The Journal of
Sports Medicine and Physical Fitness 2021;61(6):
857–66. https://doi.org/10.23736/S0022-4707.21.
11443-4.

31. Xie Y, Liu S, Chen XJ, Yu HH, Yang Y, Wang W. Effects of Exercise on Sleep Quality and Insomnia in
Adults: A Systematic Review and Meta-Analysis of
Randomized Controlled Trials. Frontiers in Psychiatry 2021;12:664499. https://doi.org/10.3389/fpsyt.
2021.664499.

32. Baglioni C, Bostanova Z, Bacaro V, et al.
A Systematic Review and Network Meta-Analysis
of Randomized Controlled Trials Evaluating the Evidence Base of Melatonin, Light Exposure, Exercise,
and Complementary and Alternative Medicine for
Patients with Insomnia Disorder. Journal of Clinical
Medicine 2020;9(6). https://doi.org/10.3390/
jcm9061949.

33. Passos GS, Poyares DL, Santana MG, Tufik S,
Mello MT. Is exercise an alternative treatment for
chronic insomnia? Clinics (Sao Paulo) 2012;67(6):
653–60.

34. Rubio-Arias JA, Marin-Cascales E, Ramos-
Campo DJ, Hernandez AV, Perez-Lopez FR. Effect
of exercise on sleep quality and insomnia in
middle-aged women: A systematic review and
meta-analysis of randomized controlled trials. Matur-
itas 2017;100:49–56. https://doi.org/10.1016/j.
maturitas.2017.04.003.

35. Hartescu I, Morgan K, Stevinson CD. Psychomotor
Performance Decrements following a Successful

Physical Activity Intervention for Insomnia. Behavioral Sleep Medicine 2020;18(3):298–308. https://doi.org/10.1080/15402002.2019.1578774.

36. Yeung WF, Lai AY, Ho FY, et al. Effects of Zero-time Exercise on inactive adults with insomnia disorder: a pilot randomized controlled trial. Sleep Medicine 2018;52:118–27. https://doi.org/10.1016/j.sleep.2018.07.025.

37. Kyle SD, Aquino MR, Miller CB, et al. Towards standardisation and improved understanding of sleep restriction therapy for insomnia disorder: A systematic examination of CBT-I trial content. Sleep Medicine Reviews 2015;23:83–8. https://doi.org/10.1016/j.smrv.2015.02.003.

38. Edinger JD, Wohlgemuth WK, Radtke RA, Coffman CJ, Carney CE. Dose-response effects of cognitive-behavioral insomnia therapy: a randomized clinical trial. Sleep 2007;30(2):203–12. https://doi.org/10.1093/sleep/30.2.203.

39. Edinger JD, Wohlgemuth WK, Radtke RA, Marsh GR, Quillian RE. Cognitive behavioral therapy for treatment of chronic primary insomnia: a randomized controlled trial. JAMA 2001;285(14):1856–64. https://doi.org/10.1001/jama.285.14.1856.

40. Kyle SD, Morgan K, Spiegelhalder K, Espie CA. No pain, no gain: an exploratory within-subjects mixed-methods evaluation of the patient experience of sleep restriction therapy (SRT) for insomnia. Sleep Medicine 2011;12(8):735–47. https://doi.org/10.1016/j.sleep.2011.03.016.

41. Youngstedt SD, O'Connor PJ, Dishman RK. The effects of acute exercise on sleep: a quantitative synthesis. Sleep 1997;20(3):203–14.

42. Puetz TW, O'Connor PJ, Dishman RK. Effects of chronic exercise on feelings of energy and fatigue: a quantitative synthesis. Psychological Bulletin 2006;132(6):866–76. https://doi.org/10.1037/0033-2909.132.6.866.

43. Loy BD, O'Connor PJ, Dishman RK. Effect of Acute Exercise on Fatigue in People with ME/CFS/SEID: A Meta-analysis. Medicine and Science in Sports and Exercise 2016;48(10):2003–12. https://doi.org/10.1249/MSS.0000000000000990.

44. Youngstedt SD, Elliott JA, Kripke DF. Human circadian phase-response curves for exercise. Journal of Physiology 2019;597(8):2253–68. https://doi.org/10.1113/JP276943.

45. Riemann D, Spiegelhalder K, Feige B, et al. The hyperarousal model of insomnia: a review of the concept and its evidence. Sleep Medicine Reviews 2010;14(1):19–31.

46. Dressle RJ, Feige B, Spiegelhalder K, et al. HPA axis activity in patients with chronic insomnia: A systematic review and metaanalysis of case-control studies. Sleep Medicine Reviews 2022;62:101588.

47. Parsons CE, Zachariae R, Landberger C, et al. How does cognitive behavioural therapy for insomnia work? A systematic review and meta-analysis of mediators of change. Clin Psychol Rev 2021;86:102027. https://doi.org/10.1016/j.cpr.2021.102027.

48. Kalmbach DA, Cheng P, Arnedt JT, et al. Treating insomnia improves depression, maladaptive thinking, and hyperarousal in postmenopausal women: comparing cognitive-behavioral therapy for insomnia (CBTI), sleep restriction therapy, and sleep hygiene education. Sleep Medicine 2019;55:124–34.

49. Li Y, Vgontzas AN, Fernandez-Mendoza J, et al. Effect of trazodone versus cognitive-behavioural treatment on high- and slow-frequency activity during non-rapid eye movement sleep in chronic insomnia: a pilot, randomized clinical trial. J Sleep Res 2021;30(5):e13324.

50. Youngstedt SD, Dishman RK, Cureton KJ, et al. Does body temperature mediate anxiolytic effects of acute exercise? J Appl Physiol 1993;74(2):825–31.

51. Raglin JS, Morgan WP. Influence of exercise and quiet rest on state anxiety and blood pressure. Medicine and Science in Sports and Exercise 1987;19(5):456–63.

52. Irwin MR, Olmstead R, Carrillo C, et al. Cognitive behavioral therapy vs. Tai Chi for late life insomnia and inflammatory risk: a randomized controlled comparative efficacy trial. Sleep 2014;37(9):1543–52.

53. Irwin MR, Olmstead R, Breen EC, et al. Cognitive behavioral therapy and tai chi reverse cellular and genomic markers of inflammation in late-life insomnia: a randomized controlled trial. Biol Psychiatry 2015;78(10):721–9.

54. Kothari V, Cardona Z, Chirakalwasan N, et al. Sleep interventions and glucose metabolism: systematic review and meta-analysis. Sleep Medicine 2021;78:24–35.

55. Espie CA, Emsley R, Kyle SD, et al. Effect of Digital cognitive behavioral therapy for insomnia on health, psychological well-being, and sleep-related quality of life: a randomized clinical trial. JAMA Psychiatry 2019;76(1):21–30.

56. Belleville G, Cousineau H, Levrier K, et al. Meta-analytic review of the impact of cognitive-behavior therapy for insomnia on concomitant anxiety. Clin Psychol Rev 2011;31(4):638–52.

57. Shimodera S, Watanabe N, Furukawa TA, et al. Change in quality of life after brief behavioral therapy for insomnia in concurrent depression: analysis of the effects of a randomized controlled trial. J Clin Sleep Med 2014;10(4):433–9.

58. Lack L, Sweetman A. Diagnosis and treatment of insomnia Comorbid with obstructive sleep apnea. Sleep Medicine Clinics 2016;11(3):379–88.

59. Abd El-Kader SM, Al-Jiffri OH. Aerobic exercise affects sleep, psychological wellbeing and immune

system parameters among subjects with chronic primary insomnia. Afr Health Sci 2020;20(4): 1761–9.

60. Rouleau CR, Horsley KJ, Morse E, et al. The association between insomnia symptoms and mood changes during exercise among patients enrolled in cardiac rehabilitation. J cardiopulmonary Rehabil Prev 2015;35(6):409–16.

61. Barham WT, Buysse DJ, Kline CE, et al. Sleep health mediates the relationship between physical activity and depression symptoms. Sleep & breathing = Schlaf & Atmung 2021. https://doi.org/10.1007/s11325-021-02496-9.

62. Janssen H, Venekamp LN, Peeters GAM, et al. Management of insomnia in sleep disordered breathing. Eur Respir Rev 2019;28(153). https://doi.org/10.1183/16000617.0080-2019.

63. Iftikhar IH, Kline CE, Youngstedt SD. Effects of exercise training on sleep apnea: a meta-analysis. Lung 2014;192(1):175–84.

64. Kline CE, Crowley EP, Ewing GB, et al. The effect of exercise training on obstructive sleep apnea and sleep quality: a randomized controlled trial. Sleep 2011;34(12):1631–40.

65. Morin CM, Hauri PJ, Espie CA, et al. Nonpharmacologic treatment of chronic insomnia. An American Academy of Sleep Medicine review. Sleep 1999; 22(8):1134–56.

66. Beaver WL, Wasserman K, Whipp BJ. A new method for detecting anaerobic threshold by gas exchange. J Appl Physiol 1986;60(6):2020–7.

67. Goldberg L, Elliot DL, Kuehl KS. Assessment of exercise intensity formulas by use of ventilatory threshold. Chest 1988;94(1):95–8.

Wearable Device-Delivered Intensive Sleep Retraining as an Adjunctive Treatment to Kickstart Cognitive-Behavioral Therapy for Insomnia

Darah-Bree Bensen-Boakes, B.Psyc (Hons)[a], Tara Murali, B.Psyc (Hons)[b], Nicole Lovato, PhD[a], Leon Lack, PhD[a], Hannah Scott, PhD[a],*

KEYWORDS

- Insomnia • Sleep onset insomnia • Intensive sleep retraining
- Cognitive-behavioral therapy for insomnia • Consumer sleep technology • Sleep tracker
- Wearable device

KEY POINTS

- Intensive Sleep Retraining is a technique that is as effective at resolving insomnia symptoms as first-line behavioral techniques but achieves these benefits after a single day rather than multiple weeks.
- The multiple rapid sleep onsets experienced during the treatment session, compelled by increasing homeostatic sleep drive and circadian-optimal times for sleep, are thought to extinguish conditioned insomnia for patients with sleep initiation difficulties.
- Wearable technology has been developed to enable the administration of Intensive Sleep Retraining in the home environment, improving its accessibility to insomnia patients.
- Pending further testing with this technology across various populations, Intensive Sleep Retraining may be used as an adjunctive therapy to produce rapid sleep improvements.

INTRODUCTION

Given that a large proportion of insomnia patients are unable to access and/or unwilling to engage in traditional cognitive-behavioral therapy for insomnia (CBT-I), alternative viable treatment options are needed. Such options would ideally be highly efficacious, simple to administer at home, and inexpensive. Presently, behavioral therapies (eg, sleep restriction and stimulus control therapies) are the most efficacious components of CBT-I,[1,2] and can be administered at home for relatively low cost via digital CBT-I.[3] If there is a downside to this treatment modality, it is the time (4 to 8 weeks) and time on task (one session per week plus daily diaries) required. Intensive Sleep Retraining is a potential alternative to CBT-I which requires only one treatment session. Moreover, Intensive Sleep Retraining is a potential adjunct to boosting the short-term efficacy of CBT-I. This review will discuss the research to date on Intensive Sleep Retraining, its administration via sleep monitoring technology, as well as why and how it could be used to kick-start insomnia treatment.

[a] Flinders Health and Medical Research Institute: Sleep Health, Flinders University, GPO Box 2100, Adelaide, SA, 5001; [b] College of Education, Psychology and Social Work, Flinders University, GPO Box 2100, Adelaide, SA, 5001
* Corresponding author.
E-mail address: hannah.scott@flinders.edu.au

Sleep Med Clin 18 (2023) 49–57
https://doi.org/10.1016/j.jsmc.2022.09.006
1556-407X/23/© 2022 Elsevier Inc. All rights reserved.

Intensive Sleep Retraining: Its Development and Efficacy

Intensive Sleep Retraining had its unlikely beginnings in basic science research into circadian rhythms. Lack and colleagues[4] assessed whether changes in skin temperature around the sleep onset period were due to the initiation of sleep or temperature rhythm variations using a modified constant routine protocol. Good sleepers were given a sleep opportunity every 30 min over 45 h whereby they were awoken shortly after entering NREM Stage 1 sleep (N1 sleep) on each sleep opportunity. During this procedure, participants soon started experiencing very rapid sleep latencies, presumably because the little duration of sleep that they were experiencing with each sleep attempt was not enough to satiate homeostatic sleep drive. Gradisar and colleagues[5] extended this research by comparing changes in skin temperature between good sleepers and people with insomnia using the same protocol administered over 26 h. Notably, the participants with insomnia fell asleep rapidly during this procedure at a similar rate to the good sleepers. The combination of a high homeostatic sleep drive during phases of the circadian rhythm where alertness is reduced (ie, around 4 to 5 am for most people and during the "post-lunch dip") was thought to have reduced sleep latencies in both groups. The authors hypothesized that this procedure might be therapeutic, and thus began more than two decades of research into Intensive Sleep Retraining.

Intensive Sleep Retraining was subsequently tested in two pilot studies. The first study was by Lack and Baraniec.[6] Ten people with sleep onset insomnia were recruited, as it was presumed that the reduction of sleep latencies experiencing during the procedure would be most therapeutic for the insomnia subtype which frequently experience lengthy sleep latencies. Following Intensive Sleep Retraining, participants experienced large decreases in sleep latency (pretreatment = 75 min, posttreatment = 32 min) and increases in total sleep time (pretreatment = 312, posttreatment = 397 min) relative to pretreatment.[6] The second pilot study was by Harris and colleagues,[7] who recruited 17 sleep onset insomnia patients and implemented the same treatment procedure: a sleep opportunity, or "sleep trial", every 30 min for 24 to 28 h (about 50 sleep trials on average). Participants who typically took 70 min to fall asleep each night experienced an average sleep latency of 6.9 min (SD = 3.6) during this experimental procedure.[7] Similar to the prior pilot study,[6] following Intensive Sleep Retraining, participants experienced large

decreases in sleep latency (pretreatment: mean [M] = 69.94 [SD = 35.38]; posttreatment: M = 39.46 [SD = 18.71]) and increases in total sleep time (pretreatment: M = 317.20 [SD = 80.19]; posttreatment: M = 381.76 [SD = 68.90]) after the single treatment session.[7] Further, there were small decreases in wake after sleep onset (pretreatment: M = 87.49; [SD = 63.03]; posttreatment: M = 59.46 [SD = 53.88]) and increases in sleep efficiency (pretreatment: M = 62.44 [SD = 15.85]; posttreatment: M = 75.71 [SD = 13.64]). These promising findings suggested that the short sleep latencies experienced during laboratory-based Intensive Sleep Retraining resulted in reduced latencies and improved sleep in the home environment.

Following the pilot studies, a randomized controlled trial was conducted by Harris and colleagues[8] to test the efficacy of Intensive Sleep Retraining. This trial randomized 80 participants with sleep onset insomnia to four conditions: Intensive Sleep Retraining alone, 4 weeks of in-person stimulus control therapy (SCT), the combination (Intensive Sleep Retraining followed by 4 weeks of SCT) versus a sleep hygiene control group. All three active treatment groups showed large and significant improvements in sleep following treatment compared with the control group.[8] The reductions in sleep latency were comparable between the Intensive Sleep Retraining (pretreatment: M = 61.41 [SD = 25.21]; posttreatment: M = 38.41 [SD = 16.24], d = 0.61) and SCT (pretreatment: M = 68.33 [SD = 44.04]; posttreatment: M = 38.94 (SD = 29.39], d = 0.78) conditions.[8] This was despite Intensive Sleep Retraining taking place over a single 26-h session versus 4 weeks of therapy: a much more rapid treatment for comparable benefit to sleep. In addition, the effects after this one session were maintained at the final follow-up timepoint for the study, six months after treatment. Importantly, the combination of these therapies was particularly efficacious, with larger decreases in sleep latency (pretreatment: M = 60.79 [SD = 42.79]; posttreatment: M = 24.70 [SD = 12.83], d = 0.96) and increases in total sleep time (pretreatment: M = 357.41 [SD = 65.61]; posttreatment: M = 411.91 [SD = 50.91], d = 0.83).[8] These findings heralded Intensive Sleep Retraining as a step forward in the rapid treatment of insomnia using behavioral techniques.[9]

Why Is Intensive Sleep Retraining Efficacious?

We hypothesize three potential mechanisms (acting alone or in combination) that are driving the efficacy of Intensive Sleep Retraining.[10,11]

First, the increase in homeostatic sleep drive resulting from the near-total sleep deprivation during the treatment session. This high sleep drive results in long recovery sleeps on the 1 to 2 nights following treatment, which may be a cognitively therapeutic experience for individuals with insomnia who report fearing that they can never, and have lost the ability to, sleep well. Participants frequently reported anecdotally the best sleep in "years" on the recovery nights. Insomnia patients also report fear about losing sleep. The experience of sleep loss during Intensive Sleep Retraining does not seem to be aversive, as no participants in the three earlier mentioned studies withdrew before completing the procedure.[6–8] Participants mainly reported strong feelings of sleepiness, which may have been a welcomed long sought experience. However, the high sleep drive alone would not explain the observed improvements in sleep that are sustained for at least six months following Intensive Sleep Retraining.

Second, the feedback received about the experience of falling asleep may partially resolve sleep-state misestimation. Feedback is repeatedly given to the individual about whether they had fallen asleep with each sleep trial during Intensive Sleep Retraining. This may result in individuals learning to associate the sensations and mental activity of "light" sleep with sleep rather than wakefulness. Research has shown that even good sleepers awoken from light sleep sometimes (30%) guess they had been awake rather than asleep, whereas those with chronic insomnia usually (70%) claim they had been awake.[12] However, if this was to occur, it would presumably also lead to reduced wake after sleep onset following Intensive Sleep Retraining, which seems to only reduce by a small degree.[7,8]

Third, the extinguishing of conditioned insomnia through repeated experiences of attempting sleep coupled with rapid sleep onsets. Individuals with sleep onset insomnia may associate the bedroom and attempting sleep with extended wakefulness due to repeated episodes of struggling to fall asleep. Over time, this may condition individuals to experience anxiety and sleeplessness when trying to fall asleep, as hypothesized under the updated "4P" (predisposing, precipitating, perpetuating, and Pavlovian conditioning) model for insomnia.[13,14] The frequent, rapid sleep onsets experienced during Intensive Sleep Retraining are manifested by high homeostatic sleep drive and circadian propensity for sleep. These rapid sleep onsets may extinguish said conditioned insomnia, and instead, 'retrain' participants to fall asleep rapidly when attempting sleep; hence, the name of this therapy. In this sense, Intensive Sleep Retraining effectively results in dozens of rapid sleep onset experiences over just one night instead of once per night over several weeks with SCT.[10]

Out of the three potential mechanisms, the latter appears to be the most likely mechanism to explain most cases in the efficacy trials to date, as significant reductions in cognitive sleep anticipatory anxiety were observed.[7] Further research is required to determine the mechanism(s) responsible for the efficacy of Intensive Sleep Retraining as this could help maximize the benefits of this, and other, insomnia treatments.

Implementation Barriers to Intensive Sleep Retraining

Although the efficacy trials to date indicate that laboratory-based Intensive Sleep Retraining is an effective rapid treatment for insomnia, the laborious and resource-heavy process makes this procedure unsustainable to implement routinely in practice.[11] The in-laboratory procedure requires sleep technicians to setup and monitor polysomnography recording to determine sleep onset and arouse patients from sleep during each sleep trial. These resources are costly, especially as Intensive Sleep Retraining is not covered under public health systems or private health insurance, so the patient would need to bear the full cost. These resources are also inaccessible to many individuals who reside in rural and remote locations, or in locations where the available sleep clinics do not offer this service. Consequently, Intensive Sleep Retraining was a viable treatment option for few individuals, until now.

To overcome these barriers to implementation, individuals would ideally be able to self-administer Intensive Sleep Retraining in their homes. Potential benefits to home-based Intensive Sleep Retraining include the reduced reliance on overstretched healthcare resources, reduced cost, and increased convenience for patients. Aside from these benefits, administration of Intensive Sleep Retraining in the home environment may also be more efficacious than the laboratory-based modality given the proposed mechanisms of action. If Intensive Sleep Retraining predominantly treats insomnia by extinguishing the conditioned insomnia around attempting sleep and retraining people to fall asleep more quickly in its place, then conducting this learning process in the environment in which insomnia typically occurs would presumably be most effective. Therefore, the administration of Intensive Sleep Retraining in the home environment was a worthwhile endeavor for both efficacy and practicality reasons. Nonetheless, home-based Intensive Sleep Retraining comes with its own barriers to implementation.

Enabling Home-Based Intensive Sleep Retraining with Technology

It is important to note that the aforementioned RCT data are limited to one large RCT in a sleep laboratory setting, and an RCT of the same scale is yet to be conducted entirely outside of the sleep laboratory (ie, in the participant's home) testing THIM-administered Intensive Sleep Retraining. At the time, there was no sleep monitoring technology available that had the capability necessary to help individuals administer Intensive Sleep Retraining in the home. The devices that existed for at-home sleep monitoring either failed to achieve a high enough degree of accuracy for sleep onset detection (eg, wrist-worn sleep trackers),[15] or could not detect sleep onset in real-time to subsequently wake the user promptly enough (eg, EEG headbands).[16] In response, a phone application was invented called "Sleep On Cue."[17] This application would detect behavioral responses to stimuli to estimate sleep onset: a method that dated back to the early beginnings of sleep stage measurement in the 1950s.[18] The phone application required users to shake the phone when they heard an auditory stimulus (tone sound played by the phone) that occurred approximately every 30 s. When the user failed to respond to two consecutive stimuli, it was assumed that they had fallen asleep, so the application would emit a high-intensity alarm sound to wake them. After a brief break, the user would be able to attempt sleep again while monitored by the phone application; thus, undergoing the Intensive Sleep Retraining procedure.

Preliminary work found that this procedure was accurate enough at estimating sleep onset (after about 2 min of N1 sleep) for the purpose of Intensive Sleep Retraining.[18] However, this procedure came with limitations.[19] The method of behavioral response (holding and shaking the phone) was cumbersome and may have caused arousal and disruption to the process of initiating sleep. In addition, the tone stimuli were difficult to calibrate to a volume level that the participant could reliably detect when awake but not be too alerted by it when attempting sleep. On occasion, the earphones that were used to deliver the stimuli at a reliable volume would detach from the ear, meaning that participants would not hear the tone stimuli, or the resulting high-intensity alarm, and sleep through the remaining duration of the procedure without intervention.[19] Although these limitations impeded the administration of Intensive Sleep Retraining, the ease of this procedure for individuals to detect sleep onset and undergo sleep trials was promising.

A wearable device called THIM was created specifically to mobilize Intensive Sleep Retraining for home administration.[20,21] Like Sleep On Cue, THIM relies upon individuals tapping their finger in response to vibrations emitted from the device about every 30 s. As such, THIM can accurately estimate sleep onset (within 30–60 s of polysomnography derived N1 sleep onset)[21] so that individuals can be woken up after only briefly initiating sleep. Rather than determining sleep onset through complex polysomnography-based devices that are often relatively expensive and cumbersome to use, even those that are developed for 'simplified home use', individuals could instead use simple, inexpensive behavioral response-based devices like THIM to detect sleep onset accurately.

These technological developments meant that individuals could self-administer Intensive Sleep Retraining feasibly and reliably in the home environment. The wearable-device administered procedure is as follows (as depicted in **Fig. 1**). THIM connects to the THIM smartphone application via Bluetooth for setup. The device is worn on the user's index finger of their dominant hand. During Intensive Sleep Retraining, THIM administers low-intensity tactile vibrations and users respond by tapping their index finger on which they are wearing THIM onto their thumb. A detected tap response indicates that they are awake. If responses to two consecutive vibrations are not detected, the device assumes that the user has fallen asleep, and a subsequent higher intensity vibration is administered to wake up the individual. After a brief break (about 5 min), the device administers an intense vibration to indicate that the user can attempt another sleep trial. This process continues until the pre-specified duration of Intensive Sleep Retraining is complete, after which the high-intensity vibrations cease, and the user can sleep uninterrupted until the wake-up alarm in the morning. THIM-administered Intensive Sleep Retraining deviates from the traditional method by collapsing the 50+ sleep onsets across one 26-h session (one every 30 min) into a much briefer (and likely more favorable) overnight session with very brief breaks between sleep trials.[10,19] Thus, THIM has the potential to enable the successful and practical administration of Intensive Sleep Retraining for anyone in the home environment.

Intensive Sleep Retraining as a Stand-Alone or an Adjunct Therapy?

These efficacy studies showed that Intensive Sleep Retraining may be a viable stand-alone treatment. However, better results may be

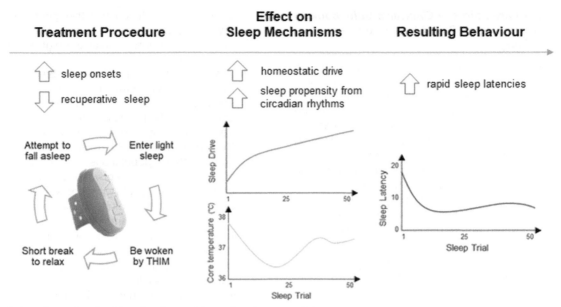

Fig. 1. The cycle of THIM-administered intensive sleep retraining.

obtained when used as an adjunct to CBT-I. Although Intensive Sleep Retraining produced similar benefits to sleep and daytime impairment outcomes as four weeks of SCT, the combination was most effective. In terms of treatment responsiveness between the Intensive Sleep Retraining, SCT, and the combined treatment conditions, 46.7%, 37.5%, and 61.1% of participants were categorized as "treatment responders," respectively.[8] In addition, Intensive Sleep Retraining resulted in similar improvements in dysfunctional beliefs and sleep self-efficacy to SCT,[8] but targeted therapies to directly treat these cognitions would be desirable as this may prevent relapse. Accordingly, where CBT-I is also available and appropriate to administer, it is recommended that Intensive Sleep Retraining is used as an adjunctive therapy (eg, before SCT). The effects of administering Intensive Sleep Retraining before Sleep Restriction Therapy or Intensive Sleep Retraining combined with both SCT and Sleep Restriction Therapy is unknown, as these treatment combinations are untested. Nonetheless, under the many circumstances where CBT-I is improbable to administer, Intensive Sleep Retraining may be useful as a stand-alone therapy to rapidly treat sleep initiation difficulties.

Further, Intensive Sleep Retraining may serve best as a technique to boost the short-term efficacy of CBT-I. In the randomized controlled trial, Intensive Sleep Retraining provided a substantial 'kick-start' to treatment, such that reductions in sleep latency and wake after sleep onset emerged earlier (week 1 versus week 4 for SCT) and were of

a greater magnitude at posttreatment compared with either treatment alone.[8] Because patients in the combined condition completed Intensive Sleep Retraining first, they commenced SCT with less severe sleep onset difficulties than pretreatment. Accordingly, patients recovered faster. In addition, adherence to traditional behavioral therapies can be problematic, especially outside of the research setting.[22] Kick-starting treatment with Intensive Sleep Retraining means that patients may be better equipped to adhere and cope with the behavioral components of CBT-I, resulting in reductions in symptoms beyond what can be achieved with either treatment alone. Thus, the combination of Intensive Sleep Retraining and CBT-I (with the therapies occurring in that order) may result in substantially greater treatment efficacy and adherence. This idea will be tested in future research studies into Intensive Sleep Retraining.

Moreover, if the efficacy of Intensive Sleep Retraining is due to its ability to resolve conditioned insomnia, then adjunctive therapies which target other specific perpetuating factors may increase treatment efficacy even further. For example, the use of circadian rhythm therapies during insomnia treatment with patients who have circadian disruption (ie, circadian misalignment) may lead to the greater resolution of sleeping difficulties.[23] We propose that Intensive Sleep Retraining is used in a similar manner: as an adjunctive therapy for those with significant sleep initiation difficulties who may exhibit conditioned insomnia.

Clinics Care Points: a Clinician's Guidebook to Delivering Home-Based Intensive Sleep Retraining

The following section serves as guide for clinicians in the administration of Intensive Sleep Retraining with patients. Please note that this information is based on the current state of evidence at the time of writing and more research is needed to test the efficacy of Intensive Sleep Retraining across different populations and modes of delivery. Information pertaining to appropriate usage, dosage, administration, contraindications, and side effects of Intensive Sleep Retraining are summarized in **Table 1**. Frequently asked questions are answered further below. The hope is that this information will prepare clinicians to administer Intensive Sleep Retraining appropriately with insomnia patients and improve the efficacy of the sleep medicine community's clinical practices.

Frequently asked questions

Q1: The patient does experience sleep initiation difficulties, but predominately experiences sleep maintenance difficulties. Is Intensive Sleep Retraining potentially beneficial for them?

A1: Intensive Sleep Retraining may be beneficial in this case for treating the sleep initiation difficulties–assuming that the sleep initiation difficulties are substantial enough to justify a targeted intervention–but it is unlikely that the sleep maintenance difficulties would resolve after this procedure. In prior studies, patients often experienced both sleep onset and sleep maintenance insomnia yet tended to experience only small reductions in time awake after sleep onset (WASO) after Intensive Sleep Retraining. Intensive Sleep Retraining followed by further treatment (eg, sleep restriction therapy) would likely be required to address both sleep difficulties.

Q2: The patient has a comorbid sleep disorder (eg, obstructive sleep apnea). Is Intensive Sleep Retraining potentially beneficial for them?

A2: Although this determination would need to be made on a case-by-case basis, Intensive Sleep Retraining may be used for some patients with comorbid sleep disorders to treat sleep initiation difficulties. In the specific case of mild obstructive sleep apnea, close monitoring of daytime sleepiness would be necessary on the day following Intensive Sleep Retraining (eg, avoiding driving and other potentially dangerous activities before they get recovery sleep) as sleepiness would likely be elevated even further than the high levels at baseline.

It is important to note that Intensive Sleep Retraining may be contraindicated in the presence of other comorbidities. More specifically, the necessary near-total sleep deprivation component to Intensive Sleep Retraining will not be tolerated well by some patient populations. For example, such levels of sleep deprivation are not recommended for people with Bipolar Disorder because it can precipitate manic episodes. Likewise, some patients may not be willing to experience heightened sleepiness in the 1-2 days following Intensive Sleep Retraining due to commitments such as work or caring responsibilities.

If the patient is currenting taking any medications to treat their sleep disorder(s), this should be considered before undergoing Intensive Sleep Retraining. Intensive Sleep Retraining may not be recommended in combination with some medications, for instance, those that promote drowsiness. If the medication is being used to 'help sleep', withdrawal options should be considered if Intensive Sleep Retraining is used.

Q3: What are the known side effects to Intensive Sleep Retraining?

A3: The most common side effect to Intensive Sleep Retraining is increased sleepiness during the treatment session and for 1–2 days following treatment. The increased sleepiness may also result in impaired daytime performance. For this reason, patients should be cautioned to not drive or operate heavy machinery until they feel recovered. There are no known long-term side effects to Intensive Sleep Retraining.

Q4: How can I best prepare patients on what to expect with Intensive Sleep Retraining?

A4: Before Intensive Sleep Retraining, it is recommended that clinicians discuss with patients 1) the experience of the procedure and 2) plan for the logistics for its administration. First, patients should be prepared for the high levels of sleepiness experienced during Intensive Sleep Retraining. These feelings can be re-framed as a positive experience, as it indicates that the treatment is working as the sleepiness will help them fall asleep more quickly. Patients should also be prepared for the sensations of waking from light sleep, which often does

Table 1
The clinician's guide to administering intensive sleep retraining

	Recommendation
Indication and Usage	Intensive Sleep Retraining has only been tested with patients reporting *sleep initiation difficulties* ($\geq$30-min sleep latencies) who meet diagnostic criteria for Insomnia Disorder.
	Intensive Sleep Retraining may serve as a stand-alone treatment, but is most efficacious when used immediately before the commencement of behavioral therapies during CBT-I.
Dosage	Best evidence to date shows its efficacy when a sleep trial is administered every 30 min for 24 h. Only one treatment session was required.
	Recent preliminary work suggests that 30–40 sleep trials condensed into an overnight session (<12 h) can still significantly reduce insomnia symptoms.[19]
Administration	Best evidence to date was conducted using laboratory-based Intensive Sleep Retraining.
	Emerging evidence about the feasibility of wearable device-administered Intensive Sleep Retraining in the home environment suggests that this modality may be similarly efficacious to the laboratory-based method.
Contraindications	With patients for whom acute sleep restriction/total sleep deprivation is not recommended, such as people with Bipolar Disorder.
Side Effects	Increased sleepiness during and immediately after treatment. Patients should refrain from driving/operating heavy machinery in the 1–2 days after treatment until they feel recovered and have experienced an adequate recovery sleep.

Please note: Information presented in this table is based on the current state of evidence at the time of writing and is subject to change based on new information about Intensive Sleep Retraining.

not feel like 'real sleep'. Asking patients to focus on what they recall immediately before being woken up during Intensive Sleep Retraining may help them realize that they were indeed asleep, reduce their frustration arising from the misestimation that they had not yet fallen asleep, and contribute to a therapeutic effect.

Second, the logistics about undergoing a night of Intensive Sleep Retraining should be considered. As this technique is ideally undertaken in the patient's bedroom, the sleeping arrangements for any bed partners should be considered as their sleep will likely be disrupted and they may therefore want to sleep elsewhere on that treatment night (if possible). In addition, activities undertaken during the brief break in-between sleep trials should be determined before the Intensive Sleep Retraining session. It is recommended that they leave the bedroom in-between each sleep trial if they are able to do so, in which case, quiet activities should be undertaken. Research is currently being undertaken to determine whether breaks in-between trials are necessary for efficacious results.

Q5: When should patients undergo Intensive Sleep Retraining?

A5: Intensive Sleep Retraining should be scheduled before a rest day (ie, not a workday or when they have other substantial responsibilities) and should commence at their typical bedtime. If the patient has caring responsibilities, a night should be chosen when another person can undertake this role.

Q6: The patient reports trepidation about repeatedly being woken up. How can I address these concerns?

A6: As discussed in A3, the high levels of sleepiness experienced during Intensive

Sleep Retraining can be re-framed into a positive experience as it reinforces that the re-conditioning process is likely working. In addition, the acute levels of sleepiness will not harm them, especially when the procedure is scheduled for when they do not have substantial responsibilities the following day. To date, 100+ patients have undergone the Intensive Sleep Retraining procedure in the prior efficacy studies, without any adverse events: this may be reassuring to patients. Further, the acute sleepiness experience is also likely to lead to long-term benefits: the short-term pain for long-term gain is a worthwhile trade-off for the substantial proportion of patients who have experienced insomnia for many years.

Q7: What should patients do/not do during the breaks in-between sleep trials?

A7: It is recommended that patients leave the bedroom (if possible) and undertake quiet activities during the breaks in-between sleep trials, such as reading, completing crosswords, and watching television in dim light. These activities should not be so uninteresting/unengaging as to potentially allow patients to fall asleep in-between trials. Patients may also wish to toilet during breaks to avoid interrupting a sleep trial. Activities that are potentially too alerting should be avoided, such as gaming, social media, and exercising. Bright light and consuming food and caffeine should also be avoided.

Q8: The patient underwent the Intensive Sleep Retraining procedure and is convinced that they were awake throughout the session (ie, did not sleep at all). What could this indicate?

A8: This may occur when patients have a substantial sleep-state discrepancy. As discussed in A3, patients may view the sensation of light sleep as more like with wake than sleep. Asking patients to attempt to recall their thoughts immediately before the end of the sleep trial may help them realize that they were asleep.

Q9: Can the patient sleep during the day (ie, nap) immediately following the nighttime intensive sleep retraining?

A9: We suggest they plan activities during the day following their nighttime training and avoid a daytime nap/sleep. Instead, we suggest they go to bed 1 to 2 h earlier than normal for their following nighttime recovery sleep. It may well be the case that the experience of a robust recovery sleep the following night is a therapeutic element of the intensive sleep re-training procedure.

SUMMARY

Although efficacious for treating sleep initiation difficulties as a stand-alone therapy, Intensive Sleep Retraining may be particularly useful as an adjunctive treatment to CBT-I. With clear treatment gains emerging after just one treatment session, Intensive Sleep Retraining may serve as a kickstart to therapy to reduce insomnia severity and encourage greater adherence to other behavioral treatments during CBT-I. To date, only one large RCT on Intensive Sleep Retraining has been conducted in a sleep laboratory setting. With technological developments enabling its feasible administration outside of the sleep laboratory, Intensive Sleep Retraining is now a viable option for the substantial number of insomnia patients for whom this technique would previously have been inaccessible. With these new technologies, avenues for future research have the potential to include an RCT conducted entirely in the participant's home using devices such as Sleep On Cue or THIM. With research aiming to maximize the effectiveness of Intensive Sleep Retraining, the hope is that the sleep medicine community will adopt this efficacious technique into their clinical practice.

CLINICS CARE POINTS

- Intensive Sleep Retraining has only been tested with patients reporting sleep initiation difficulties. It is unknown if the treatment will be efficacious for patients with other sleep difficulties.

- Increased sleepiness during and in the 1 to 2 days following treatment is the main known side effect to Intensive Sleep Retraining.

- Intensive Sleep Retraining may serve as a stand-alone treatment but is more efficacious when used before the commencement of behavioral therapies during the course of cognitive-behavioral therapy for insomnia.

DISCLOSURE

L. Lack is a shareholder of Re-Time Pty Ltd. H. Scott and N. Lovato were previously consultants to Re-Time Pty Ltd. L. Lack and H. Scott have a patent regarding the THIM device. D-B. Bensen-Boakes, TM and NL have no conflicts of interest to disclose.

REFERENCES

1. Maurer LF, Schneider J, Miller CB, et al. The clinical effects of sleep restriction therapy for insomnia: a meta-analysis of randomised controlled trials. Sleep Med Rev 2021;58:101493.

2. Edinger JD, Arnedt JT, Bertisch SM, et al. Behavioral and psychological treatments for chronic insomnia disorder in adults: an American Academy of Sleep Medicine clinical practice guideline. J Clin Sleep Med 2021;17(2):255–62.

3. Zachariae R, Lyby MS, Ritterband LM, et al. Efficacy of internet-delivered cognitive-behavioral therapy for insomnia - a systematic review and meta-analysis of randomized controlled trials. Sleep Med Rev 2016; 30:1–10.

4. Lack L, Gradisar M. Acute finger temperature changes preceding sleep onset over a 45-h period. J Sleep Res 2002;11(4):275–82.

5. Gradisar M, Lack L, Wright H, et al. Do chronic primary insomniacs have impaired heat loss when attempting sleep? Am J Physiol Regul Integr Comp Physiol 2006;290(4):R1115–21.

6. Lack L, Baraniec M. Intensive sleep onset training for sleep onset insomnia. Sleep 2002;25(Abstract Supplement):A478–9.

7. Harris J, Lack L, Wright H, et al. Intensive sleep retraining treatment for chronic primary insomnia: a preliminary investigation. article. J Sleep Res 2007; 16(3):276–84.

8. Harris J, Lack L, Kemp K, et al. A randomized controlled trial of intensive sleep retraining (ISR): a brief conditioning treatment for chronic insomnia. Article Sleep 2012;35(1):49–60.

9. Spielman AJ, Glovinsky PB. What a difference a day makes. Sleep 2012;35(1):11–2.

10. Lack L, Scott H, Lovato N. Intensive sleep retraining treatment of insomnia. Sleep Med Clin 2019;14(2): 245–52.

11. Lack L, Scott H, Micic G, et al. Intensive sleep retraining: from bench to bedside. Brain Sci 2017; 7(4). https://doi.org/10.3390/brainsci7040033.

12. Mercer JD, Bootzin RR, Lack LC. Insomniacs' perception of wake instead of sleep. Sleep 2002; 25(5):559–66.

13. Perlis ML, Giles DE, Mendelson WB, et al. Psychophysiological insomnia: the behavioural model and a neurocognitive perspective. J Sleep Res 1997; 6(3):179–88.

14. Perlis M, Shaw P, Cano G, et al. Models of insomnia. In: Kryger MH, Roth T, Dement WC, editors. Principles and practice of sleep medicine. 5th edn ed. Philadelphia, PA: Elsevier Saunders; 2011. p. 850–65.

15. Haghayegh S, Khoshnevis S, Smolensky MH, et al. Accuracy of wristband Fitbit models in assessing sleep: systematic review and meta-analysis. J Med Internet Res 2019;21(11):e16273.

16. Scott H, Lack L, Lovato N. A systematic review of the accuracy of sleep wearable devices for estimating sleep onset. Sleep Med Rev 2019;49:101227.

17. MicroSleep. Sleep on cue-research application (Version 1.1). Available at: https://itunes.apple.com/au/app/sleep-on-cue/id829583727?mt=8. Accessed April 18, 2017.

18. Scott H, Lack L, Lovato N. A pilot study of a novel smartphone application for the estimation of sleep onset. J Sleep Res 2018;27(1):90–7.

19. Mair A, Scott H, Lack L. Intensive sleep retraining treatment for insomnia administered by smartphone in the home: an uncontrolled pilot study. J Clin Sleep Med 2022;18(6):jcsm. 9892.

20. Scott H, Lovato N, Lack L. The development and accuracy of the THIM wearable device for estimating sleep and wakefulness. Nat Sci Sleep 2021;13:39.

21. Scott H, Whitelaw A, Canty A, et al. The accuracy of the THIM wearable device for estimating sleep onset latency. J Clin Sleep Med 2021;17(5):jcsm. 9070.

22. Kyle SD, Morgan K, Spiegelhalder K, et al. No pain, no gain: an exploratory within-subjects mixed-methods evaluation of the patient experience of sleep restriction therapy (SRT) for insomnia. Sleep Med 2011;12(8):735–47.

23. Evans MA, Hasler BP. Adapting cognitive behavioral therapy for insomnia. Elsevier; 2022. p. 63–95. CBT-I for patients with phase disorders or insomnia with circadian misalignment.

Mindfulness as an Adjunct or Alternative to CBT-I

Jason C. Ong, PhD[a,b,*], David A. Kalmbach, PhD[c,d]

KEYWORDS

• Insomnia • Sleep • Mindfulness • Meditation • MBI • MBSR • Cognitive arousal • Metacognition

KEY POINTS

- Clinical trial data support mindfulness-based interventions (MBIs) to alleviate self-reported symptoms of insomnia and cognitive arousal, the latter being central to the development of insomnia and its chronicity.
- Mindfulness practice is hypothesized to reduce nighttime hyperarousal (a key treatment mechanism) by targeting a metacognitive level of sleep-related arousal. Emerging studies on the mechanisms of mindfulness provide some preliminary support for this model and the association between the mindfulness principles of awareness, nonreaction, and self-compassion and sleep quality.
- For the treatment of insomnia, MBIs should be explored as both an adjunct therapy (including integrated approaches combining mindfulness practice with behavioral sleep strategies) and an alternative to cognitive behavioral therapy for insomnia (CBT-I).
- MBIs may be preferential for certain patient populations, including pregnant women, hypnotic-dependent insomnia patients, individuals with multiple morbidities, and for patients who do not sufficiently respond to CBT-I.
- As mindfulness practice does not target sleep disturbances directly, MBIs may be effective strategies to prevent the development of chronic insomnia disorder in at-risk individuals, including those with intermittent acute insomnia episodes.

INTRODUCTION

Insomnia disorder is a highly prevalent sleep disorder affecting about 10% to 18% of adults.[1,2] Although cognitive behavioral therapy for insomnia (CBT-I) has emerged as the first-line treatment, approximately 40% to 60% of patients do not achieve full remission from insomnia.[3–5] Given the high prevalence of insomnia, there remains a need to enhance the armamentarium of treatments to effectively reduce the public health burden of this sleep disorder.

One promising approach comes from mindfulness meditation, a practice that is aimed at promoting mind–body regulation. Mindfulness-based interventions (MBI) are multiweek experiential training programs that teach mindfulness meditation as a health behavior to regulate emotion and cope with stressful conditions. MBIs have been used as an adjunct or an alternative to CBT-I, and there is increasing evidence to support its effectiveness in reducing insomnia symptoms. Additional evidence is starting to provide some insights about how mindfulness might be effective in managing insomnia, leading to some indications about who might benefit from a mindfulness approach compared with other insomnia treatments.

[a] Department of Neurology, Center for Circadian and Sleep Medicine, Northwestern University Feinberg School of Medicine, 710 N. Lake Shore Dr, Chicago, IL 60625, USA; [b] Behavioral Sleep Medicine, Nox Health, 5000 Research Court, Suite 500, Suwanee, GA 30024, USA; [c] Thomas Roth Sleep Disorders Center, Henry Ford Health System, 39450 W 12 Mile Road, Novi, Detroit, MI 48377, USA; [d] Department of Pulmonary & Critical Care and Sleep Medicine, Wayne State University School of Medicine, Detroit, MI, USA
* Corresponding author: Center for Circadian and Sleep Medicine, Department of Neurology, Northwestern University Feinberg School of Medicine, 710 N. Lake Shore Dr, Chicago, IL 60625.
E-mail address: jong@noxhealth.com

Sleep Med Clin 18 (2023) 59–71
https://doi.org/10.1016/j.jsmc.2022.09.002
1556-407X/23/© 2022 Elsevier Inc. All rights reserved.

This article presents an overview of the use of mindfulness practices for insomnia. First, a definition of mindfulness concepts and a brief history of mindfulness interventions are reviewed. Next, we present the theoretic models regarding how mindfulness is hypothesized to reduce insomnia symptoms along with research findings related to these concepts. Subsequently, we summarize the evidence for the effectiveness of mindfulness for insomnia from randomized controlled trials (RCTs) and reviews along with a discussion of the findings. Based on current findings, we discuss clinical considerations for using mindfulness as an adjunct or an alternative to CBT-I, noting specific populations or situations in which mindfulness could be advantageous over CBT-I or other approaches.

MINDFULNESS CONCEPTS AND HISTORY OF MBIs

Mindfulness can be defined as bringing focus to the present experience by *intentionally* paying *attention* to the present moment with an *attitude* that is accepting and nonjudging.[6,7] This intentional awareness of mindfulness involves a cognitive process known as metacognition, which refers to an awareness or knowledge of one's own thoughts and feelings and has been referred to as "thinking about thinking." By focusing on each moment in this particular way, there is a shift from an outcome-oriented thinking (eg, actions to relieve stress) to a process-oriented approach (eg, observing that one is stressed). This metacognitive shift is posited to reduce emotional distress by changing the *relationship with* stress rather than changing the environment or source of stress.[6–8] Much like any skill, this focus requires regular practice, which is achieved through meditations that are part of a lifestyle. Key mindfulness concepts and practices are summarized in **Table 1**.

Mindfulness concepts originated from Buddhist philosophy as a means of reducing suffering and relieving stress. In Western societies, these concepts have been taught in classes or group-based courses known as MBIs to manage stress and improve the quality of life. MBIs are experiential programs led by an experienced mindfulness teacher, who leads guided meditations and group-based discussions about mindfulness principles. Participants are encouraged to establish a meditation practice for further training on how to embody these principles. With regular practice, participants can apply these mindfulness principles to adaptively cope with stress and skillfully regulate emotional distress.

Developed by Jon Kabat-Zinn,[6] mindfulness-based stress reduction (MBSR) is the seminal MBI with a widespread impact and popularity that has been adopted in clinics and hospitals around the world to help patients cope with a variety of mental and physical health issues. Although MBSR is seen as the standard MBI, it was developed to be a general program and not designed to address symptoms of specific conditions. As a result, several adaptations to MBSR have modified the types of meditations or the content of the group-based discussions to specifically address certain medical and psychiatric conditions. Mindfulness-based cognitive therapy (MBCT) was developed specifically to prevent the relapse of depression,[9] and other adaptations have been made to address substance abuse relapse[10] and menopausal symptoms.[11] Tai Chi Chih (TCC) is a physical activity program focusing on Tai Chi as a form of mindful movement. Although the structure of TCC is somewhat different from the traditional structure of MBSR, TCC is similar to other MBIs in that it teaches the principle of mindfulness through the practice of meditation. Moreover, Tai Chi is sometimes included as a movement meditation in MBSR programs. A substantial body of evidence supports the effectiveness of MBIs on reducing psychological symptoms, particularly symptoms of depression and anxiety, and improving the quality of life in several chronic medical (eg, cancer, heart disease) and psychiatric conditions (eg, depression, generalized anxiety disorder).[12–14] Further supporting MBIs for a wide range of patient populations, there are no known side effects to practicing mindfulness meditation. Therefore, they merit consideration as a viable alternative or adjunctive treatment to traditional treatments such as pharmacotherapy or psychotherapy.

Several mindfulness programs have been used to improve sleep health and reduce sleep disturbances (**Table 2**). General MBIs, such as MBSR and mindful awareness practices (MAP), have been used for primary and comorbid insomnia. MBCT has been used in people with depression and insomnia. Mindfulness-based therapy for insomnia (MBTI) was developed specifically for chronic insomnia disorder[15,16] and mindfulness and relaxation training for insomnia (MRTI) was developed for postmenopausal women with insomnia.[17] Recent studies have also examined online delivery of mindfulness programs, either through a mobile app[18] or a digital mindfulness program for insomnia.[19] Finally, one study examined the use of mindfulness-based relapse prevention on hypnotic use.[20] Below, we examine the theory and evidence for the mechanisms of using

Table 1 Key mindfulness concepts and meditation practices	
Mindfulness Concepts	**Description and Relevance for Insomnia**
Metacognition	Awareness or knowledge of one's own cognitive process or a meta-level governing of thoughts and beliefs. A metacognitive shift involves a reorientation of mental processes rather than a direct change of the mental contents or thoughts themselves. This shift is hypothesized to reduce cognitive arousal by changing the relationship with sleep-related thoughts rather than putting an increased effort to sleep (ie, spending time in bed trying to sleep).
Awareness	Purposeful attention to the present moment without judgment or attachment. Awareness of the mental and physical states associated with readiness for sleep are important in the context of insomnia.
Non-Reacting	Acceptance or acknowledgment of the present-moment experience without the need to immediately fix the problem or make it better. This is an aspect of metacognitive shifting that is hypothesized to reduce cognitive arousal and reduce maladaptive behavioral coping in people with insomnia.
Non-Attachment	Experience of the present moment while letting go of the desire for a particular outcome is seen as the pathway to relieve the distress that comes with that attachment. Attachment to the need for sleep is hypothesized to lead to cognitive arousal and rigid expectations that is characteristic of insomnia.
Self-Compassion	Act of kindness toward oneself, especially during difficult or stressful situations. The practice of mindfulness to manage cognitive and emotional distress is seen as an act of self-compassion.
Mindfulness Meditations	**Description**
Mindful Breathing	Quiet meditation focusing on the breath while observing sensations in the body while breathing.
Mindful Sitting	Quiet meditation to observe thoughts, sensations, and feelings arising in the mind and body.
Body Scan	Quiet meditation to bring awareness to a part of the body and letting go in a sequence through the body.
Walking Meditation	Movement meditation to bring awareness to the body in motion by walking with a slow, deliberate pace.
Hatha Yoga	Movement meditation to bring awareness to the body in motion through light stretching and gentle yoga postures.
Tai Chi	A form of movement meditation using sequences of slow, controlled movements.

Note. The mindfulness concepts presented in this table consist of principles and core tenets that are typically taught in mindfulness-based interventions (MBIs) and are considered to be most relevant to insomnia and sleep disturbances. Similarly, the mindfulness meditations presented in this table consist of the most common meditations taught in MBIs. The actual concepts and meditations taught might vary across different MBIs depending on how specific or general the program is designed.

mindfulness for insomnia followed by a brief review of the current evidence on treatment outcomes for using MBIs to improve sleep.

HOW DOES MINDFULNESS REDUCE INSOMNIA SYMPTOMS?

The predominant etiologic model of insomnia posits that hyperarousal of the autonomic nervous system (ANS) is the central pathophysiological mechanism that results in chronic sleep disturbance and daytime fatigue.[21,22] This can involve an overactivation of the sympathetic nervous system across sleep and wakefulness[23] or a failure to dearouse in the transition from wake to sleep.[24,25] ANS dysregulation can be triggered from cognitive activity (eg, racing thoughts at bedtime or maladaptive sleep-related thoughts) and behavioral factors (eg, spending excessive time and effort in bed). The "3-P model" uses these concepts to explain how predisposing and precipitating factors converge to create insomnia symptoms with the perpetuating factors maintaining the insomnia symptoms in the transition from acute insomnia to a chronic insomnia disorder.[26]

Given the prominence of hyperarousal in the pathophysiology of insomnia, MBIs are seen as a viable treatment option because they are hypothesized to reduce arousal through the self-regulation effects achieved from mindfulness practices. Applying the concept of metacognition to the hyperarousal hypothesis of insomnia, the metacognitive model of insomnia posits that mindfulness can reduce hyperarousal by targeting a metacognitive level of sleep-related arousal.[8] *Metacognitive arousal* consists of how individuals relate to their thoughts about sleep (eg, absorption of the sleep problem and the attachment to sleep need). This is in contrast to the traditional notion of *cognitive arousal*, which refers to heightened cognitive activity directly related to the inability to sleep (eg, sleep-interfering thoughts at night). In this model, metacognitive arousal can amplify the negative valence and attachment to the specific thoughts about sleep. For instance, the sleep-interfering thought, "I'm not going to sleep tonight," creates cognitive arousal in bed at night. A rigid attachment to this sleep-interfering thought creates an additional layer of metacognitive arousal, characterized by absorption in the sleep problem and difficulty letting go of catastrophic sleep-related thoughts, which ultimately perpetuates the insomnia.

Mindfulness practices aim to increase awareness of mental and physical states that are present when experiencing insomnia symptoms. This allows a shift in metacognition in response to these symptoms and promotes an adaptive, mindful stance characterized by balanced appraisals, cognitive flexibility, equanimity, and recommitment to values. For example, rather than ruminating on the outcome-oriented thought, "I am not going to sleep tonight," mindfulness practices encourage a shift toward a process-oriented thought, "I am not sleeping at this moment, but let's take this moment by moment and see how the night unfolds." Maintaining this mindful stance allows sleep-related arousal (ie, sleep-focused rumination, sleep effort) to subside and normal sleep patterns to reemerge. Over time, this approach is posited to have downstream effects on reducing cognitive arousal. In contrast to cognitive therapy or CBT-I, which typically uses cognitive restructuring techniques to challenge maladaptive thoughts that lead to subsequent maladaptive behaviors, mindfulness-based approaches teach patients to change their relationship with cognition and emotions by developing an objective, compassionate, and inquisitive approach to cognition and emotions. This change in perspective can promote improved self-regulation, increased cognitive and emotional flexibility, and decreased experiential avoidance.[27]

Studies examining the mechanisms of mindfulness are beginning to emerge. A study examining the relationship between metacognition for insomnia (assessed using the Metacognition Questionnaire – Insomnia [MCQ-I]), trait hyperarousal, and presleep cognitive arousal found that insomnia-specific metacognition was associated with trait hyperarousal, which is a predisposing factor of insomnia.[28] Moreover, the insomnia-metacognitive activity may mediate the effects of trait hyperarousal on presleep cognitive arousal, which is often a perpetuating factor in chronic insomnia. Further work is needed to confirm these findings, but they provide support for the plausibility of the metacognitive model of insomnia[8] and how it might connect with a traditional model of insomnia (ie, 3-P Model).

Other studies have examined how specific principles of mindfulness might impact sleep quality (**Table 1**). A longitudinal study conducted in a clinical sample of 127 colorectal cancer survivors found significant and positive indirect effects of awareness and nonreaction on self-reported sleep quality via symptom burden and emotional distress.[29] Using a measure of self-compassion with daily diaries for sleep and stress over 2 weeks, Hu and colleagues[30] found that self-compassion buffered the impact of stress on sleep latency. Specifically, those who were low in self-compassion showed an increase in sleep onset latency with an increasing number of stressors reported during the day, whereas individuals high in self-compassion reported no change in sleep onset latency regardless of the number of stressors reported during the day. Additionally, a recent cross-sectional study examining the relationship between self-compassion, sleep quality, and the 3-P model of insomnia found that low self-compassion is a potential risk factor for poor sleep quality.[31] Importantly, the relationship between self-compassion and sleep quality was mediated by anxiety about sleep. Taken together, these findings indicate that awareness, nonreaction, and self-compassion are key principles of mindfulness that appear to be involved in improving sleep quality through reducing or buffering the impact of emotional distress and cognitive arousal. However, it should be noted that these studies were not conducted on people with insomnia, so it remains unclear if these findings would translate to insomnia disorders.

In addition to psychological mechanisms, studies have examined biological mechanisms

Table 2
List of Mindfulness-Based Interventions (MBIs) used for Insomnia and Sleep Disturbances

Name		Description
MBSR	Mindfulness-Based Stress Reduction	Seminal 8-wk program teaching mindfulness in a general context. MBSR has been used in primary and comorbid insomnia.
MAP	Mindful Awareness Practices	6-wk program similar to MBSR that teaches mindfulness concepts in a general context.
MBCT	Mindfulness-Based Cognitive Therapy	8-wk program adapted from MBSR designed to prevent the relapse of depression. MBCT has been used for people with depression and insomnia.
MBTI	Mindfulness-Based Therapy for Insomnia	8-wk program integrating mindfulness with behavioral strategies for insomnia.
MBRP	Mindfulness-Based Relapse Prevention	8-wk program using mindfulness practices for reducing cravings in people with addictions. MBRP has been used with hypnotic-dependent insomnia.
MRTI	Mindfulness and Relaxation Therapy for Insomnia	8-wk program designed to address insomnia in postmenopausal women
TCC	Tai Chi Chih	Physical activity program using repetitious, nonstrenuous slow mindful movements. TCC has been used in older adults with insomnia as well as comorbid insomnia.

based on the concept that mindfulness is hypothesized to reduce physiologic hyperarousal. Currently, there are only a few studies that have used polysomnography (PSG) to measure objectively measured sleep with MBIs. At the macroarchitecture level, the available evidence indicates a pretreatment to post-treatment reduction in total wake time, although the effect size is relatively small.[15,32] Given that high-frequency electroencephalography activity in the beta and gamma range during NREM has been posited to be a marker of cortical hyperarousal and physiologic correlate of insomnia, 2 studies have examined changes in sleep microarchitecture in people who received MBI. Contrary to expectations, Britton and colleagues reported an increase in the NREM gamma range (25–40 Hz) activity along with an increase in stage 1 and decrease in slow-wave sleep in people with insomnia and depression who received MBCT.[32] In primary insomnia, Goldstein and colleagues[33] found significant increases in NREM beta (16–25 Hz) power from baseline to post-treatment and 6-month follow-up in people who received MBSR or MBTI, and increased gamma (25–40 Hz) power at 6-month follow-up for the MBTI group. In both studies, the increased cortical arousal was in contrast to the reductions in self-reported

insomnia symptoms. These paradoxic findings have led to a hypothesis that the practice of mindfulness meditation might lead to a state of "calm alertness" characterized by relating to physiologic arousal in a nonreactive manner, thereby allowing a perception of improvements in sleep despite indications of hyperarousal.[33] This hypothesis requires further testing in larger samples and highlights the importance of collecting more biological and physiologic measures in future MBI treatment studies.

CURRENT EVIDENCE BASE FOR USING MINDFULNESS TO IMPROVE SLEEP/INSOMNIA

The evidence base for using mindfulness meditation to improve sleep has grown considerably with many RCTs testing the efficacy and effectiveness of MBIs and several reviews and meta-analyses,[34–39] summarizing the aggregate findings. The reader is directed to these reviews for details related to specific findings and limitations of the literature. In this section, we provide a brief summary of the findings while focusing our discussion on specific studies that directly compared mindfulness with CBT-I as a treatment for insomnia.

In general, the current evidence indicates that MBIs can be effective for improving self-reported outcomes on sleep quality and insomnia whereas the data on objective measures of sleep are very limited and currently indicate only small treatment effects on reducing total wake time. The most consistent effects are seen in global measures of sleep quality and insomnia severity, such as the Pittsburgh sleep quality index (PSQI) and the insomnia severity index (ISI).[36,38] With respect to the effects on specific self-reported sleep parameters, MBIs appear to reduce total wake time at night, but the effects on other sleep parameters are smaller and more variable.[37] Although these findings are encouraging, previous reviews have commented on several important limitations when interpreting these findings. First, there is considerable heterogeneity and inconsistency across samples with regard to criteria for insomnia or sleep disturbance, making it difficult to evaluate mindfulness as an alternative intervention for insomnia disorder.[36] In addition, there is a lack of specificity in isolating the effects of mindfulness meditation such that other factors (eg, behavioral components, social support, nonspecific factors) could account for the observed treatment effects.[36] Finally, the rigor of the RCTs have been criticized for methodological issues including lack of blinding and insufficient adherence measures for the practice of meditation. These issues could contribute to bias, particularly as the strongest effects have been observed in the self-reported measures of sleep and insomnia symptoms. Indeed, the few studies that have used PSG and actigraphy have found relatively small effects on objectively measured sleep parameters.[35] Given that insomnia is diagnosed based on self-report, one might conclude that thus far MBIs have shown a greater impact on reducing insomnia symptoms compared with improving sleep per se.

Within this literature, only a few studies have directly compared mindfulness with CBT-I. Garland and colleagues[40] conducted a noninferiority trial comparing MBSR versus CBT-I for individuals with cancer and insomnia. Using a noninferiority margin of 4 points on the ISI, MBSR was inferior to CBT-I at post-treatment, but noninferior to CBT-I 3 months after treatment. Irwin and colleagues[41] conducted a noninferiority trial comparing TCC versus CBT-I in breast cancer survivors with insomnia. TCC was noninferior at post-treatment and follow-up, and insomnia remission rates were non-inferior between TCC (37.9%) and CBT-I (46.2%).

In a secondary analysis focusing on cognitive outcomes, Ong and colleagues[42] found that MBTI was noninferior to an 8-week behavior therapy for insomnia (BT-I) on self-reported measures of sleep effort, beliefs and attitudes about sleep, trait hyperarousal, and fatigue. Finally, a study examined the additive effects of mindfulness techniques following CBT-I[43] in which participants with an insomnia disorder received a 4-session CBT-I followed by random assignment to a 4-session cognitive therapy (CT) or a 4-session MBI immediately or after a 4-week delay. CT and MBI both enhanced CBT-I effects on insomnia symptoms and sleep quality relative to control, but no differences between CT and MBI were observed.

In general, these studies confirm that CBT-I should remain a first-line treatment for insomnia but also provide some evidence that MBIs could merit consideration as a treatment option for insomnia. In people with primary insomnia disorders, MBIs appear to be capable of reducing insomnia symptoms along with reduction in cognitive arousal that are consistent with the hypothesized mechanisms of mindfulness. However, it remains unknown how mindfulness practice compares with the cognitive component of CBT-I on cognitive arousal or metacognition. In people with comorbid insomnia and cancer, it appears that empirically supported MBIs (eg, MBSR, TCC) could be a viable alternative to CBT-I. However, more comparative effectiveness studies between MBIs and CBT-I are needed to determine whether these approaches have differing effectiveness for different insomnia subtypes (eg, sleep onset vs sleep maintenance, presence of comorbid mental illness).

USING MINDFULNESS FOR INSOMNIA: HOW, WHEN AND FOR WHOM?

If MBIs or mindfulness practice are to be considered a treatment option for insomnia, should it be an adjunct or an alternative to CBT-I? Which patients are likely to benefit from a mindfulness-based approach versus CBT-I? Are there other potential uses for mindfulness practice in the context of insomnia? Based on the theoretic considerations and empirical evidence reviewed above, we provide suggestions for how MBIs could fit into the armamentarium of tools for insomnia and sleep disturbances. First, we consider situations in which mindfulness could be used as an adjunct to CBT-I or as an alternative to CBT-I. Second, we consider certain populations or conditions when MBIs might be appropriate.

Using Mindfulness as an Adjunct to CBT-I

Given that CBT-I is generally regarded as the first-line treatment, it would be reasonable to consider if mindfulness could be used to enhance CBT-I as a complementary or adjunctive treatment. This scenario includes programs that have integrated mindfulness practices with CBT-I components (eg, stimulus control, sleep restriction), such as MBTI,[15,16] or using mindfulness as an adjunctive treatment following a course of CBT-I.[43] The primary rationale for taking this approach is based upon the hypothesis that cognitive arousal—particularly refractory symptoms amid treatment failure—is difficult to treat, and high levels of rumination and worry are linked to poor therapy prognosis.[44] MBIs appear to be well-suited for reducing cognitive arousal by targeting metacognitive processes underlying the arousal. Clinical trial data indicate that MBIs are not only efficacious for insomnia but also substantially reduce cognitive arousal symptoms central to the insomnia experience. Indeed, multiple studies suggest that integrating mindfulness into behavioral therapy for insomnia augments treatment effects on cognitive arousal in this patient population.[15,42,45] It is worth highlighting that compared with standard MBSR, an integrated approach, such as MBTI, has shown superior reductions in insomnia severity over time without diluting the impact of reducing cognitive arousal.[15]

Another possibility would be to use mindfulness as a second-line treatment for those who do not achieve clinical benefits from CBT-I. The rationale for this sequential approach comes from findings in the literature that elevation in residual self-reported cognitive arousal at post-treatment is a potential marker of nonresponse to treatment. Notably, standard CBT-I produces modest effects on cognitive arousal despite reduction of these symptoms serving as an important mechanism by which cognitive-behavioral intervention alleviates insomnia.[46,47] Emerging evidence suggests that refractory cognitive arousal is a primary barrier to adequate treatment response to CBT-I. Patients who respond poorly to CBT-I report continued high levels of nighttime cognitive arousal *after treatment* relative to patients who respond favorably to CBT-I.[48,49] Importantly, cognitive arousal levels are high and do not differ between CBT-I responders and nonresponders *before treatment* in these studies. Thus, the refractory nature of these symptoms for treatment-resistant patients is not revealed until after CBT-I failure. These findings give credence to the notion that MBIs may serve as effective second-line treatment options for insomnia patients who do not achieve clinical benefits from standard CBT-I, particularly for patients who attribute their insomnia to a racing mind despite

intervention. Although not designed to address this hypothesis, the study by Wong and colleagues[43] serves as an example of how the sequential use of mindfulness following CBT-I could enhance treatment effects.

Mindfulness as an Alternative Treatment to CBT-I

Given that the current state-of-the-science has not found that MBIs are superior to CBT-I in any studies, there does not appear to be evidence to support the use of MBIs over CBT-I as the primary treatment option for insomnia. However, an argument could be made to consider MBIs as an alternative to CBT-I in situations in which CBT-I has limited success, remains untested, or is unavailable to patients. One potential use for mindfulness practices could be to prevent chronic insomnia for people with recurring episodes of acute insomnia. As stress is often a precipitating factor for insomnia, mindfulness practices could provide tools to address the underlying emotion dysregulation/cognitive arousal before it becomes a rigid pattern that is typically seen in chronic insomnia. The behavioral components of CBT-I are limited as a prevention strategy as they require some degree of sleep disturbance in order to implement behavior change. For example, sleep restriction requires a reduction in time in bed to reduce nocturnal total wake time. Consequently, this technique might be inappropriate for preventing onset in people with recurrent acute insomnia (a risk factor for chronic insomnia) who are otherwise asymptomatic. In this scenario, mindfulness practices could be introduced between episodes of insomnia to improve sleep health and prevent chronic insomnia.

Although MBIs have not been as potent as CBT-I on treatment outcomes in most studies, participants still achieve significant reductions in insomnia symptoms in most studies. Therefore, receiving an MBI could still provide benefits for patients who may not have access to specialty behavioral sleep medicine services. The proliferation of MBI programs delivered in-person and via synchronous telehealth (ie, live videoconferencing) along with the popularity of mindfulness apps in the consumer digital health space highlight the opportunity for using MBIs at the population level. Indeed, a recent review found promising evidence that virtual MBIs (delivered via telehealth or web-based app) improved sleep quality relative to controls.[50]

Another potential use of MBIs would be to reduce hypnotic use in those with hypnotic-dependent insomnia. CBT-I has also been used in this context with some success,[51–53] but some patients with hypnotic-dependent insomnia do not experience significant sleep disturbance while taking their medications, which can make it difficult to implement CBT-I for reasons similar to the situation described above with acute insomnia. However, it is worth noting that hyperarousal plays a central role in hypnotic use among individuals with insomnia disorder,[54] thereby suggesting that MBIs may be useful for reducing hypnotic use by alleviating arousal. One study examined the use of a mindfulness-based relapse prevention (MBRP) program to facilitate hypnotic withdrawal and showed promising evidence that MBRP can reduce insomnia severity and potentially reduce hypnotic use.[20] Further research is needed to evaluate the use of MBIs in these situations, but they can serve as examples for MBIs as a viable alternative to CBT-I.

Mindfulness in Specific Populations

In addition to these possibilities, there could be specific populations in whom a mindfulness approach might be a better fit than CBT-I. These include conditions in which acceptability of CBT-I is limited, the use of sleep restriction might be contraindicated, or the use of stimulus control raises questions about patient safety. These issues with CBT-I open the door for other approaches such as MBIs. Below, we offer suggestions based on the theoretic aspects and empirical evidence reviewed above for specific populations and clinical conditions when MBIs could be used as an alternative or an adjunct to CBT-I.

Sleep Disturbances in Women. Insomnia is more prevalent among women compared with men, and sleep disturbances are often worse during pregnancy and menopause. Furthermore, the use of complementary and alternative approaches, including MBIs, are common among women, particularly among those who are younger and have a higher level of education.[55] In fact, women are overrepresented in clinical trials testing MBIs for insomnia at a ratio of about 2:1 (women:men), suggesting that mindfulness practices are more popular among women than men. There is also evidence of a potential match between the symptom profile of elevated cognitive arousal among women with insomnia and the putative targets of MBIs.[56] For these reasons, mindfulness approaches could be well-suited to address sleep disturbances among women. Two specific events related to women's health merit further discussion: pregnancy and menopause.

Pregnancy and anticipation of childbirth and having a new infant can contribute to difficulties

regulating stress and significant sleep disturbances. Unsurprisingly, cognitive arousal is particularly elevated at baseline in this population as pregnant women perseverate on pregnancy, childbirth, and motherhood.[57–59] As hypnotic medications are contraindicated during pregnancy, CBT-I is typically the recommended treatment. However, approximately half of pregnant women with insomnia who complete CBT-I do not adequately respond to treatment.[60–62] Investigation into predictors of nonresponse to treatment found that pregnant women with refractory cognitive arousal (ie, those with high arousal after receiving CBT-I) are 4 times less likely to remit from insomnia than patients whose arousal decreases with CBT-I.[49] Moreover, patient feedback revealed concerns about the acceptability of the behavioral strategies, with several participants describing sleep restriction and stimulus control as "too strict" and "inflexible" to follow during pregnancy and early postpartum.[49]

These findings provide an opportunity for using MBIs for pregnant women with sleep disturbances. As described above, mindfulness practices are hypothesized to reduce cognitive arousal through metacognitive processes, which could enhance treatment outcomes in this population. Unlike CBT-I, MBIs offer specific strategies for managing mind racing in bed at night, which can take the form of worrying about childbirth, mentally planning the nursery, or perseverating on the baby's wellbeing. Indeed, research data show that pregnant women low in the mindfulness state reported elevated insomnia, depression, and cognitive arousal.[63] In addition, evidence from RCTs using MBIs during pregnancy have found that relative to controls, MBIs can reduce depressed mood, worry, and pregnancy-specific anxiety, and garner high patient engagement and satisfaction.[64–66] Thus, mindfulness approaches could be received more favorably than CBT-I while also addressing a broader array of symptoms related to worry and rumination.

Despite the potential of MBIs to improve sleep in women during pregnancy, the field currently lacks rigorous testing of MBIs for prenatal insomnia.[67,68] Preliminary work has examined a mindful yoga program in pregnant women,[69] which found evidence for decreased time awake during the night and fewer awakenings when the program was initiated during the second trimester. Another study found that an 8-week MBI (Mindful Moms Training) did not improve sleep quality but did attenuate the influence of poor sleep on perceived stress.[70] RCTs using MBCT[71] and an online MBI[72] are also ongoing but have not yet reported results. Further research is also needed to provide guidance as to whether MBIs should be used as an alternative to CBT-I, or whether integrating some behavioral components into an MBI program, such as MBTI, would be optimal for pregnant women with insomnia.

In addition to pregnancy, MBIs could be used to address sleep disturbances associated with menopause. Notably, refractory cognitive arousal has been linked to inadequate CBT-I response in postmenopausal women with insomnia disorder.[48] One study examined a mindfulness and relaxation training for insomnia (MRTI) program for insomnia in postmenopausal women and found improvements in sleep quality and overall quality of life and a reduction in menopausal and vasomotor symptoms.[11] Another study using MBSR found a significant improvement in self-reported sleep quality along with a significant reduction in the degree of bother from hot flashes that was greater in MBSR compared with the wait-list control.[73] These findings suggest that MBIs are capable of reducing the emotional distress associated with hot flashes, which would be consistent with the hypothesized metacognitive effects that could explain the improvements in sleep quality. However, these findings require further confirmation in large-scale clinical trials. Still, they provide examples of specific situations in which mindfulness practices could be particularly useful for women with insomnia.

Insomnia in Multiple Chronic Conditions and Symptom Clusters. Multiple chronic conditions, also known as multimorbidity, is an increasing public health problem affecting up to 60% of adults.[74] Chronic insomnia disorder is often comorbid with other conditions such as chronic pain and mood disorders. For example, insomnia is often comorbid with chronic migraine and the etiology appears to involve a bidirectional relationship with sleep and circadian disturbances exacerbating migraine and the attempts to cope with migraine perpetuating the insomnia disorder.[75] In conditions such as cancer, insomnia is often part of a symptom cluster with fatigue, depression, and pain. Patients with insomnia who have multimorbidities often have poor treatment outcomes and experience poor health-related quality of life.[76]

In 2008, the U.S. Department of Health and Human Services launched an initiative to address the effects of multimorbidity.[77] Recommendations for interventions focused on common risk factors and inclusion of self-management or community-based intervention programs.[76] MBIs would appear to respond to these recommendations given its emphasis on self-regulation and the increasing accessibility of MBIs in community

settings or using online apps rather than healthcare systems. From a theoretic standpoint, the focus on metacognitions could hypothetically target common cognitive factors related to insomnia (sleep-related arousal), chronic pain (cognitive appraisal of pain), and mood (decentering from negative cognitive distortions). The empirical evidence reviewed earlier suggests that MBIs can improve sleep and reduce symptoms of insomnia comorbid with cancer. Another study found improvements in sleep measures for people with insomnia and depression who received MBCT.[32] It should be noted that there were several studies that did not specify insomnia or degree of sleep disturbance in the inclusion criteria, yet still found improvements in sleep as a secondary outcome. Although CBT-I could also be used in these cases, one could argue that MBIs cast a "wider net" than CBT-I given that mindfulness practices offer a broader scope of self-regulating techniques compared with CBT-I. Indeed, MBIs that are not condition-specific (ie, MBSR) have still proven effective for improving quality of life in a wide range of patient populations, thereby supporting its application for multimorbidities. Thus, an argument could be made that MBIs merit consideration as an adjunctive or alternative treatment because they target a common underlying factor that could impact a broader array of symptoms than using CBT-I alone. Further research is needed to examine the efficacy of MBIs in multiple chronic conditions as well as testing the hypothesized effect on common cognitive factors.

Insomnia across the Lifespan. MBIs could also be used to improve sleep health and treat insomnia in specific age groups across the lifespan. Given that older adults often have multimorbidities, MBIs could be an alternative to CBT-I in older adults, particularly if there are safety concerns (ie, falls) related to getting out of bed as part of stimulus control. As described earlier, several randomized controlled trials have shown evidence to support the effectiveness of MBIs in this age range.[78–80]

In contrast to adults, there is no clear first-line treatment for insomnia in children and the empirical evidence for adapting CBT-I for children is not well-established compared with the literature for adults. Some challenges include a delay in circadian rhythms, difficulty monitoring and enforcing adherence to sleep restriction and stimulus control, and the proliferation of screen time at night. Supporting mindfulness for sleep in children, one study found an increase of 74 minutes in objectively measured total sleep time in school-aged children who received a health and mindfulness curriculum for 2 years.[81]

Future Directions and Conclusions

Mindfulness is intended to serve as a self-regulation practice to manage stress and improve mental and physical health. There is now substantial evidence indicating that MBI programs can be effective for improving sleep health and reducing symptoms of insomnia, leading to considerations of how, when, and for whom these programs should be used. Consequently, there appears to be room to consider using MBIs as an adjunct or alternative treatment particularly in situations when cognitive arousal is prominent or refractory to treatment. Women with sleep disturbances during pregnancy and menopause appear to fit this profile. Mindfulness practice could also be used as a self-regulation technique to address a range of symptoms and improve quality of life in people with multimorbidities. Finally, MBIs could be considered in situations where insomnia symptoms are currently subthreshold, such as the case with hypnotic-dependent insomnia or between episodes of recurrent acute insomnia.

It should be emphasized that the suggestions presented here are based primarily on theoretic grounds with limited empirical evidence. Further research that directly addresses the issues raised (eg, is mindfulness more acceptable than CBT-I for certain populations?) or tests the sequence of using MBIs with CBT-I (eg, is MBI a viable second-line treatment for insomnia?) are required before these can be adopted as clinical guidelines or recommendations. As such, a priority for future directions is to determine who is likely to benefit from a mindfulness approach compared to CBT-I (ie, predictors of treatment response). A second priority would be to dismantle MBI packages and examine the specific effects of mindfulness meditation on sleep and recovery. This also includes questions related to the optimal amount, timing, and type of meditation (movement vs quiet meditation) for people with insomnia. Finally, questions related to the implementation science of mindfulness should be investigated. These include the use of digital or remote delivery of MBIs along with potential ways to measure adherence to meditation using wearable or tracking technology. Such research can also examine ways to increase access to both MBIs and CBT-I at the population level and test unique combinations of mindfulness and CBT-I components, promoting further understanding of how and when these tools could be used. These future directions can improve the treatment toolbox for insomnia and allow patients and clinicians to optimize treatment outcomes for insomnia.

CLINICS CARE POINTS

- Mindfulness practice and meditation can be very useful for reducing cognitive arousal in patients with insomnia, which may help alleviate insomnia or even prevents its development.

- Mindfulness as adjunct to behavioral sleep treatment (e.g., Mindfulness-based therapy for insomnia [MBTI]) may be a treatment of choice in patients with prominent worry and rumination at night.

- Many insomnia patients who fail CBT-I report high levels of residual congnitive arousal. For patients who fail CBT-I, MBIs may represent a viable second-stage therapy by addressing a critical unmet need.

REFERENCES

1. Ohayon MM. Epidemiology of insomnia: what we know and what we still need to learn. Sleep Med Rev 2002;6(2):97–111.
2. Morin CM, LeBlanc M, Daley M, Gregoire JP, Merette C. Epidemiology of insomnia: prevalence, self-help treatments, consultations, and determinants of help-seeking behaviors. Sleep Med 2006;7(2):123–30. S1389-9457(05)00195-4 [pii].
3. Morin CM, Vallières A, Guay B, et al. Cognitive behavioral therapy, singly and combined with medication, for persistent insomnia: a randomized controlled trial. JAMA 2009;301(19):2005–15.
4. Wu JQ, Appleman ER, Salazar RD, Ong JC. Cognitive behavioral therapy for insomnia comorbid with psychiatric and medical conditions: a meta-analysis. JAMA Intern Med 2015;175(9). https://doi.org/10.1001/jamainternmed.2015.3006.
5. Buysse DJ, Germain A, Moul DE, et al. Efficacy of brief behavioral treatment for chronic insomnia in older adults. Arch Intern Med 2011;171(10):887–95.
6. Kabat-Zinn J. Full catastrophe living: using the wisdom of your body and mind to face stress, pain, and illness. New York: Bantam Books; 2003.
7. Shapiro SL, Carlson LE, Astin JA, Freedman B. Mechanisms of mindfulness. J Clin Psychol 2006; 62(3):373–86.
8. Ong JC, Ulmer CS, Manber R. Improving sleep with mindfulness and acceptance: a metacognitive model of insomnia. Article. Behav Res Ther 2012; 50(11):651–60.

9. Segal ZV, Williams JMG, Teasdale JD. Mindfulness-based cognitive therapy for depression: a new approach to preventing relapse. New York: The Guilford Press; 2013.

10. Bowen S, Chawla N, Witkiewitz K. Mindfulness-based relapse prevention for addictive behaviors. Mindfulness-based treatment approaches. New York: Elsevier; 2014. p. 141–57.

11. Garcia MC, Kozasa EH, Tufik S, Mello LEA, Hachul H. The effects of mindfulness and relaxation training for insomnia (MRTI) on postmenopausal women: a pilot study. Menopause 2018;25(9): 992–1003.

12. Khoury B, Lecomte T, Fortin G, et al. Mindfulness-based therapy: a comprehensive meta-analysis. Clin Psychol Rev 2013;33(6):763–71.

13. Hofmann SG, Sawyer AT, Witt AA, Oh D. The effect of mindfulness-based therapy on anxiety and depression: a meta-analytic review. J consulting Clin Psychol 2010;78(2):169.

14. Goyal M, Singh S, Sibinga EMS, et al. Meditation programs for psychological stress and well-being: a systematic review and meta-analysis. JAMA Intern Med 2014;174(3):357–68.

15. Ong JC, Manber R, Segal Z, Xia Y, Shapiro S, Wyatt JK. A randomized controlled trial of mindfulness meditation for chronic insomnia. Article. *Sleep.* 2014;37(9):1553–63.

16. Ong JC, Manber R. Mindfulness-based therapy for insomnia. Handbook of Mindfulness-Based Programmes, Itai Ivtzan. ed., 1st edn. London: Imprint Routledge; 2019.

17. Garcia MC, Kozasa EH, Tufik S, Mello LEAM, Hachul H. The effects of mindfulness and relaxation training for insomnia (mrti) on postmenopausal women: a pilot study. Menopause 2018;25(9). https://doi.org/10.1097/GME.0000000000001118.

18. Huberty JL, Green J, Puzia ME, et al. Testing a mindfulness meditation mobile app for the treatment of sleep-related symptoms in adults with sleep disturbance: a randomized controlled trial. Plos one 2021;16(1):e0244717.

19. Kennett L, Bei B, Jackson ML. A randomized controlled trial to examine the Feasibility and preliminary efficacy of a digital mindfulness-based therapy for improving insomnia symptoms. Mindfulness 2021;12(10):2460–72.

20. Barros VV, Opaleye ES, Demarzo M, et al. Effects of mindfulness-based relapse prevention on the chronic use of hypnotics in treatment-seeking women with insomnia: a randomized controlled trial. Int J Behav Med 2021;1–12.

21. Bonnet MH, Arand DL. Hyperarousal and insomnia: state of the science. Sleep Med Rev 2010;14(1): 9–15.

22. Riemann D, Spiegelhalder K, Feige B, et al. The hyperarousal model of insomnia: a review of the concept and its evidence. Sleep Med Rev 2010; 14(1):19–31.

23. Bonnet MH, Arand DL. Hyperarousal and insomnia. Sleep Med Rev 1997;1(2):97–108.

24. Espie CA. Insomnia: conceptual issues in the development, persistence, and treatment of sleep disorder in adults. Annu Rev Psychol 2002;53:215–43.

25. Nofzinger EA, Buysse DJ, Germain A, Price JC, Miewald JM, Kupfer DJ. Functional Neuroimaging evidence for hyperarousal in insomnia. Am J Psychiatry 2004;161(11):2126–8.

26. Spielman AJ, Caruso LS, Glovinsky PB. A behavioral perspective on insomnia treatment. Psychiatr Clin North Am 1987;10(4):541–53.

27. Shapiro SL, Carlson LE, Astin JA, Freedman B. Mechanisms of mindfulness. J Clin Psychol 2006; 62(3):373–86.

28. Palagini L, Ong JC, Riemann D. The mediating role of sleep-related metacognitive processes in trait and pre-sleep state hyperarousal in insomnia disorder. Article. J Psychosomatic Res 2017;99:59–65.

29. Fong TC, Ho RT. Mindfulness facets predict quality of life and sleep disturbance via physical and emotional distresses in Chinese cancer patients: a moderated mediation analysis. Psycho-oncology. 2020;29(5):894–901.

30. Hu Y, Wang Y, Sun Y, Arteta-Garcia J, Purol S. Diary study: the protective role of self-compassion on stress-related poor sleep quality. Mindfulness 2018;9(6):1931–40.

31. Rakhimov A, Ong J, Realo A, Tang NKY. Being kind to self is being kind to sleep? A structural equation modelling approach evaluating the direct and indirect associations of self-compassion with sleep quality, emotional distress and mental well-being. Article. Curr Psychol 2022. https://doi.org/10.1007/s12144-021-02661-z.

32. Britton WB, Haynes PL, Fridel KW, Bootzin RR. Polysomnographic and subjective profiles of sleep continuity before and after mindfulness-based cognitive therapy in partially remitted depression. Psychosom Med 2010;72(6):539–48.

33. Goldstein MR, Turner AD, Dawson SC, et al. Increased high-frequency NREM EEG power associated with mindfulness-based interventions for chronic insomnia: preliminary findings from spectral analysis. J Psychosomatic Res 2019;120:12–9.

34. Wang Y-Y, Wang F, Zheng W, et al. Mindfulness-based interventions for insomnia: a meta-analysis of randomized controlled trials. Behav Sleep Med 2020;18(1):1–9.

35. Ong JC, Smith CE. Using mindfulness for the treatment of insomnia. Review. Curr Sleep Med Rep 2017;3(2):57–65.

36. Ong JC, Moore C. What do we really know about mindfulness and sleep health? Review. Curr Opin Psychol 2020;34:18–22.

37. Gong H, Ni CX, Liu YZ, et al. Mindfulness meditation for insomnia: a meta-analysis of randomized controlled trials. J Psychosom Res 2016;89:1–6.

38. Rash JA, Kavanagh VAJ, Garland SN. A meta-analysis of mindfulness-based Therapies for insomnia and sleep disturbance: Moving towards processes of change. Sleep Med Clin 2019;14(2):209–33.

39. Chen TL, Chang SC, Hsieh HF, Huang CY, Chuang JH, Wang HH. Effects of mindfulness-based stress reduction on sleep quality and mental health for insomnia patients: a meta-analysis. J Psychosom Res 2020;135:110144.

40. Garland SN, Carlson LE, Stephens AJ, Antle MC, Samuels C, Campbell TS. Mindfulness-based stress reduction compared with cognitive behavioral therapy for the treatment of insomnia comorbid with cancer: a randomized, partially blinded, noninferiority trial. J Clin Oncol : official J Am Soc Clin Oncol 2014;32(5):449–57.

41. Irwin MR, Olmstead R, Carrillo C, et al. Tai Chi Chih compared with cognitive behavioral therapy for the treatment of insomnia in survivors of breast cancer: a randomized, partially blinded, noninferiority trial. J Clin Oncol 2017;35(23):2656–65.

42. Ong JC, Xia Y, Smith-Mason CE, Manber R. A randomized controlled trial of mindfulness meditation for chronic insomnia: effects on daytime symptoms and cognitive-emotional arousal. Article Mindfulness 2018;9(6):1702–12.

43. Wong MY, Ree MJ, Lee CW. Enhancing CBT for chronic insomnia: a Randomised clinical trial of additive components of mindfulness or cognitive therapy. Clin Psychol Psychother 2016;23(5):377–85.

44. Watkins ER. Constructive and unconstructive repetitive thought. Psychol Bull 2008;134(2):163–206.

45. Ong JC, Shapiro SL, Manber R. Combining mindfulness meditation with cognitive-behavior therapy for insomnia: a treatment-development study. Article. Behav Ther 2008;39(2):171–82.

46. Espie CA, Kyle SD, Miller CB, Ong J, Hames P, Fleming L. Attribution, cognition and psychopathology in persistent insomnia disorder: outcome and mediation analysis from a randomized placebo-controlled trial of online cognitive behavioural therapy. Sleep Med 2014;15(8):913–7.

47. Cheng P, Kalmbach DA, Cuamatzi-Castelan A, Muragan N, Drake CL. Depression prevention in digital cognitive behavioral therapy for insomnia: is rumination a mediator? J Affective Disord 2020; 273:434–41.

48. Kalmbach DA, Cheng P, Arnedt JT, et al. Treating insomnia improves depression, maladaptive thinking, and hyperarousal in postmenopausal women: comparing cognitive-behavioral therapy for insomnia (CBTI), sleep restriction therapy, and sleep hygiene education. Sleep Med 2019;55:124–34.

49. Kalmbach DA, Cheng P, Roth T, et al. Examining patient feedback and the role of cognitive arousal in treatment on-response to digital cognitive-behavioral therapy for insomnia during pregnancy. Behav Sleep Med 2022;20(2):143–63.

50. Jiang A, Rosario M, Stahl S, Gill JM, Rusch HL. The effect of virtual mindfulness-based interventions on sleep quality: a systematic review of randomized controlled trials. Curr Psychiatry Rep 2021;23(9). https://doi.org/10.1007/s11920-021-01272-6.

51. Bélanger L, Belleville G, Morin CM. Management of hypnotic discontinuation in chronic insomnia. Sleep Med Clin 2009/12/01/2009;4(4):583–92.

52. Morin CM, Colecchi CA, Ling WD, Sood RK. Cognitive behavior therapy to facilitate benzodiazepine discontinuation among hypnotic-dependent patients with insomnia. Behav Ther 1995;26(4):733–45.

53. Soeffing JP, Lichstein KL, Nau SD, et al. Psychological treatment of insomnia in hypnotic-dependant older adults. Sleep Med 2008/01//2008,9(2):165–71.

54. Pillai V, Cheng P, Kalmbach DA, Roehrs T, Roth T, Drake CL. Prevalence and predictors of Prescription sleep Aid Use among individuals with DSM-5 insomnia: the role of hyperarousal. Sleep 2016; 39(4):825–32.

55. Pearson NJ, Johnson LL, Nahin RL. Insomnia, trouble sleeping, and complementary and alternative medicine: analysis of the 2002 national health interview survey data. Arch Intern Med 2006; 166(16):1775 82.

56. Hantsoo L, Khou CS, White CN, Ong JC. Gender and cognitive–emotional factors as predictors of pre-sleep arousal and trait hyperarousal in insomnia. J Psychosomatic Res 2013;74(4):283–9.

57. Martini J, Asselmann E, Einsle F, Strehle J, Wittchen H-U. A prospective-longitudinal study on the association of anxiety disorders prior to pregnancy and pregnancy-and child-related fears. J anxiety Disord 2016;40:58–66.

58. Kalmbach DA, Cheng P, Ong JC, et al. Depression and suicidal ideation in pregnancy: exploring relationships with insomnia, short sleep, and nocturnal rumination. Sleep Med 2020;65:62–73.

59. Blackmore ER, Gustafsson H, Gilchrist M, Wyman C, O'Connor TG. Pregnancy-related anxiety: evidence of distinct clinical significance from a prospective longitudinal study. J Affective Disord 2016;197: 251–8.

60. Manber R, Bei B, Simpson N, et al. Cognitive behavioral therapy for prenatal insomnia: a randomized controlled trial. Obstet Gynecol 2019;133(5): 911.

61. Felder JN, Epel ES, Neuhaus J, Krystal AD, Prather AA. Efficacy of digital cognitive behavioral therapy for the treatment of insomnia symptoms among pregnant women: a randomized clinical trial. JAMA psychiatry 2020;77(5):484–92.

62. Kalmbach DA, Cheng P, O'Brien LM, et al. A randomized controlled trial of digital cognitive

behavioral therapy for insomnia in pregnant women. Sleep Med 2020;72:82–92.

63. Kalmbach DA, Roth T, Cheng P, Ong JC, Rosenbaum E, Drake CL. Mindfulness and nocturnal rumination are independently associated with symptoms of insomnia and depression during pregnancy. Sleep Health 2020;6(2):185–91.

64. Guardino CM, Dunkel Schetter C, Bower JE, Lu MC, Smalley SL. Randomised controlled pilot trial of mindfulness training for stress reduction during pregnancy. Psychol Health 2014;29(3):334–49.

65. Goodman JH, Guarino A, Chenausky K, et al. CALM Pregnancy: results of a pilot study of mindfulness-based cognitive therapy for perinatal anxiety. Arch women's Ment Health 2014;17(5):373–87.

66. Dimidjian S, Goodman SH, Felder JN, Gallop R, Brown AP, Beck A. Staying well during pregnancy and the postpartum: a pilot randomized trial of mindfulness-based cognitive therapy for the prevention of depressive relapse/recurrence. J consulting Clin Psychol 2016;84(2):134.

67. Lucena L, Frange C, Pinto ACA, Andersen ML, Tufik S, Hachul H. Mindfulness interventions during pregnancy: a narrative review. J Integr Med 2020; 18(6):470–7.

68. Bacaro V, Benz F, Pappaccogli A, et al. Interventions for sleep problems during pregnancy: a systematic review. Sleep Med Rev 2020;50:101234.

69. Beddoe AE, Lee KA, Weiss SJ, Powell Kennedy H, Yang C-PP. Effects of mindful yoga on sleep in pregnant women: a pilot study. Biol Res Nurs 2010;11(4): 363–70.

70. Felder JN, Laraia B, Coleman-Phox K, et al. Poor sleep quality, psychological distress, and the buffering effect of mindfulness training during pregnancy. Behav Sleep Med 2018;16(6):611–24.

71. Tomfohr-Madsen LM, Campbell TS, Giesbrecht GF, et al. Mindfulness-based cognitive therapy for psychological distress in pregnancy: study protocol for a randomized controlled trial. Trials 2016;17(1):1–12.

72. Kantrowitz-Gordon I, McCurry SM, Landis CA, Lee R, Wi D. Online prenatal trial in mindfulness sleep management (OPTIMISM): protocol for a pilot randomized controlled trial. Pilot feasibility Stud 2020;6(1):1–10.

73. Carmody J, Crawford S, Salmoirago-Blotcher E, Leung K, Churchill L, Olendzki N. Mindfulness training for coping with hot flashes: results of a randomized trial. Menopause (New York, NY) 2011; 18(6):611.

74. King DE, Xiang J, Pilkerton CS. Multimorbidity Trends in United States adults, 1988–2014. J Am Board Fam Med 2018;31(4):503–13.

75. Ong JC, Park M. Chronic headaches and insomnia: Working toward a biobehavioral model. Cephalalgia 2012;32(14):1059–70.

76. Smith SM, Wallace E, O'Dowd T, Fortin M. Interventions for improving outcomes in patients with multimorbidity in primary care and community settings. Cochrane Database Syst Rev 2016;3(3):Cd006560.

77. Parekh AK, Goodman RA. The HHS Strategic Framework on multiple chronic conditions: genesis and focus on research. J Comorb 2013;3(Spec Issue):22–9.

78. Black DS, O'Reilly GA, Olmstead R, Breen EC, Irwin MR. Mindfulness meditation and improvement in sleep quality and daytime Impairment among older adults with sleep disturbances: a randomized clinical trial. JAMA Intern Med 2015;175(4):494–501.

79. Irwin MR, Olmstead R, Carrillo C, et al. Cognitive behavioral therapy vs. Tai Chi for late life insomnia and Inflammatory risk: a randomized controlled comparative efficacy trial. SLEEP 2014;37(9): 1543–52.

80. Perini F, Wong KF, Lin J, et al. Mindfulness-based therapy for insomnia for older adults with sleep difficulties: a randomized clinical trial. Article. Psychol Med 2021. https://doi.org/10.1017/S0033291721002476.

81. Chick CF, Singh A, Anker LA, et al. A school-based health and mindfulness curriculum improves children's objectively measured sleep: a prospective observational cohort study. J Clin Sleep Med 2021; 18(9):2261–71.

Acceptance and Commitment Therapy as an Adjunct or Alternative Treatment to Cognitive Behavioral Therapy for Insomnia

Kathryn S. Saldaña, PhD[a], Sarah Kate McGowan, PhD[a,b],
Jennifer L. Martin, PhD[c,d],*

KEYWORDS

• Insomnia • Acceptance • Behavioral • Treatment • Adjunctive • Cognitive-behavioral

KEY POINTS

- Increasing awareness and flexibility when experiencing insomnia symptoms helps to promote an adaptive stance toward insomnia experiences and facilitate deactivation of these same processes that hinder sleep.
- Acceptance and commitment therapy (ACT) interventions for insomnia involve targeting both sleep-interfering behaviors and cognitive arousal through incorporation of acceptance and willingness, mindfulness, cognitive defusion and self as context, and values identification and committed action.
- In ACT-based interventions for insomnia, elements of ACT are combined with evidence-based behavioral components of insomnia treatment, such as sleep restriction and stimulus control.
- Studies examining outcomes of acceptance-based interventions for insomnia demonstrate improvements in sleep outcomes and quality of life.
- Using an ACT-based approach, clinicians can individualize treatment to accommodate specific needs, such as when working with individuals with comorbid conditions and those from diverse cultures and backgrounds, or to facilitate adaptation to a patient-centered, culturally sensitive approach to insomnia treatment.

INTRODUCTION

Insomnia is a clinical disorder that affects 10% of the general population. Prevalence rates of insomnia are higher among individuals with comorbid medical and/or psychiatric conditions, older individuals, women, and military veterans. Insomnia is associated with a range of negative outcomes including reduced psychomotor performance, reduced memory consolidation, decreased work

[a] Department of Mental Health, VA Greater Los Angeles Healthcare System, 11301 Wilshire Boulevard, Los Angeles, CA 90073, USA; [b] Department of Psychiatry and Biobehavioral Sciences, David Geffen School of Medicine, University of California, Los Angeles, CA, USA; [c] VA Greater Los Angeles Healthcare System, Geriatric Research, Education, and Clinical Center, 16111 Plummer St (11E), North Hills, CA 91343, USA; [d] Department of Medicine, David Geffen School of Medicine, University of California, Los Angeles, CA, USA
* Corresponding author.
E-mail address: Jennifer.martin@va.gov

Sleep Med Clin 18 (2023) 73–83
https://doi.org/10.1016/j.jsmc.2022.09.003
1556-407X/23/Published by Elsevier Inc.

performance, and reduced quality of life (QoL).[1–4] There are strong associations between insomnia and other medical and mental health conditions such as chronic pain, depression, and anxiety.[5,6] Cognitive behavioral therapy for insomnia (CBT-I) is considered the "gold standard" treatment and is recommended as the first approach to addressing insomnia.[7] Although CBT-I has demonstrated strong efficacy and effectiveness, adherence to the treatment recommendations can be a challenge and some individuals discontinue treatment prematurely. Difficulty with treatment adherence and drop out is likely related to the counterintuitive nature of many treatment recommendations that are a part of sleep restriction and stimulus control approaches. This can lead to discouragement and reduced motivation to adhere to recommendations and complete treatment. Cognitive therapy approaches are often used to address motivation and adherence; however, some individuals find it difficult to change their thoughts related to sleep while they are still struggling with insomnia.

Acceptance and commitment therapy (ACT) is a third wave therapy that incorporates mindfulness, acceptance, and cognitive defusion to change the relationship that individuals experience toward their thoughts and emotional experience. There is some evidence that ACT and acceptance-based approaches improve sleep disturbance, and there is a strong theoretical rationale to incorporate ACT as an alternative or adjunctive approach in the treatment of insomnia. This article seeks to provide an overview of ACT-based interventions for insomnia and describe how they align and differ from CBT-I. We provide a review of the literature to date and discuss populations who may benefit from this approach.

Cognitive Behavioral Therapy for Insomnia

CBT-I is recommended as the first-line treatment of adults with insomnia.[7] CBT-I is a multicomponent therapy that is comprised of psychoeducation about sleep processes, stimulus control, sleep restriction, sleep hygiene, strategies to decrease arousal, and cognitive therapy. The 2 main behavioral components of CBT-I are stimulus control and sleep restriction. Stimulus control addresses the learned association that forms between the bed/bedroom and arousing wakeful activities (eg, watching TV, tossing and turning, worrying), which results in conditioned arousal. Within this approach, individuals are instructed to only use their beds for sleeping and sexual activity. Individuals are also instructed to get out of their beds during periods of wakefulness at night, and only return to bed when feeling sleepy. This strategy helps an individual strengthen the relationship between their bed and sleep (ie, increase their stimulus control) and thus reduce the negative effects of conditioned arousal. Sleep restriction helps to build sleep drive and consolidate sleep by limited time in bed (the sleep opportunity window) to match an individuals' total sleep time at the beginning of treatment with the goal of reducing or eliminating excessive time spent in bed awake. Once sleep quality improves, time in bed is gradually extended until the patient gets sufficient sleep. Sleep hygiene includes addressing other factors that affect sleep, including environmental conditions, use and timing of substances (eg, caffeine, alcohol, nicotine), and physical activity. Although these behavioral strategies ultimately lead to sleep consolidation and increased quality of sleep over time, their initial implementation commonly results in reduced sleep quality and total sleep time for many individuals. It should be noted that although stimulus control and sleep restriction can be efficacious in the reduction of insomnia symptoms as standalone interventions, sleep hygiene alone does not significantly reduce insomnia symptoms.[8] Counter-arousal and relaxation techniques are often included in CBT-I treatment to address the heightened arousal systems that can interfere with sleep. Cognitive therapy addresses the maladaptive thoughts and beliefs that interfere with sleep and adherence to treatment recommendations. One goal of cognitive therapy is to change or reduce the maladaptive thoughts that interfere with sleep by replacing them with more realistic and helpful thoughts.

Decades of research and meta-analyses have shown that CBT-I leads to significant improvements in subjective and objective sleep quality and quantity.[8,9] Additionally, successful completion of CBT-I is associated with decreases in depression, trauma-related mental health symptoms, chronic pain, and symptoms associated with sleep apnea.[10–13] However, not all individuals benefit from CBT-I, and many individuals struggle to adhere to treatment recommendations or discontinue treatment prematurely. Difficulty with adherence may be related to the counterintuitive nature of some treatment components (ie, sleep restriction and stimulus control) such as reducing the sleep opportunity window or getting out of bed when unable to sleep. Additionally, some studies have suggested that 14% to 40% of individuals drop out of CBT-I treatment altogether.[14] As such, adaptations to CBT-I seek to address such difficulties with treatment adherence and successful completion.

Acceptance-Based Interventions for Insomnia

ACT is one of the third wave behavioral therapies. Third wave therapies use mindfulness and acceptance as key approaches within the treatment. ACT is based on both principles that explore cognition and behavior through a holistic and context-focused perspective that allows openness and acceptance toward all psychological events, pleasant or unpleasant, or those labeled as negative or maladaptive.[15,16] ACT consists of 6 domains that are targeted in treatment: (1) Present moment focus: Use of mindfulness to become aware of present moment, without judgment, including ability to identify and tolerate inner experiences—pleasant or unpleasant; (2) Acceptance: Willingness to allow difficult inner experiences to exist, without trying to change or control them; (3) Values: Aspects of living that give meaning to one's life (eg, family, career, spirituality); (4) Cognitive defusion: Separation from and nonidentification with thoughts; (5) Self as context: Identifying observer self within that can separate from daily experiences and connect to core self; and (6) Committed action: Identification of concrete, objective goals that are values-consistent (**Fig. 1**). Through these domains, individuals change their relationship to their thoughts and emotions with an emphasis on function, rather than the form of an experience.[17]

In contrast to CBT, ACT proposes that it is not the experience of unwanted thoughts, emotions, or behaviors that cause suffering but rather the process of attempting to control, reduce, or eliminate these personal experiences that causes individuals to struggle. By engaging in experiential avoidance, individuals create more, not less, of these unwanted experiences. Furthermore, ACT theory views an individual's values as an essential foundation for goal setting in treatment. The goal of ACT, therefore, is to increase psychological and behavioral flexibility and use values to achieve a meaningful life. Individuals do so by engaging in mindfulness (eg, the act of being present in the current moment) and a variety of experiential exercises and metaphors aimed at fostering acceptance of personal experiences, disentangling who we are from our experiences, fostering a willingness to embrace inner experiences, and a commitment to making behavioral changes in accordance with one's own values.[15]

Acceptance and Acceptance and Commitment Therapy-based approaches for the treatment of insomnia

ACT is regularly used as a treatment modality for many psychiatric and medical disorders.[18,19] Thus, it is no surprise that this treatment modality is now being applied to the treatment of insomnia. Theories promoting acceptance-based interventions to treat insomnia suggest that increasing awareness and flexibility toward cognitive processes that present when experiencing insomnia symptoms may help to promote an adaptive stance toward insomnia experiences and facilitate deactivation of these same cognitive processes.[20,21] Indeed, studies have shown that ACT interventions result in significant improvements in sleep outcomes. Interventions cited in the literature include both studies that use only ACT to treat insomnia and research studies that incorporate ACT with insomnia-specific behavioral components as a more direct alternative to CBT-I; the latter approach is outlined below.

ACT-based interventions for insomnia involve targeting both sleep-interfering behaviors and cognitive arousal through a few key strategies[22,23]:

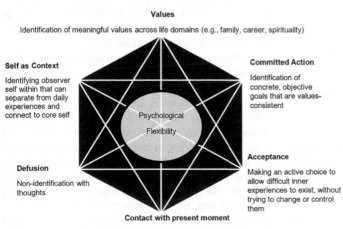

Values
Identification of meaningful values across life domains (e.g., family, career, spirituality)

Self as Context
Identifying observer self within that can separate from daily experiences and connect to core self

Committed Action
Identification of concrete, objective goals that are values-consistent

Psychological Flexibility

Defusion
Non-identification with thoughts

Acceptance
Making an active choice to allow difficult inner experiences to exist, without trying to change or control them

Contact with present moment
Use of mindfulness to become aware of present moment, without judgement, including ability to identify and tolerate inner experiences – pleasant or unpleasant

Fig. 1. This figure depicts and briefly describes each element of the Hexalfex Model of Acceptance and Commitment Therapy (ACT) Processes

1. Acquiring an accepting stance (rather than "fighting" with their insomnia) through use of willingness to experience short-term discomfort (eg, fatigue and tiredness that accompany sleep restriction and stimulus control components of insomnia treatment).
2. Increasing cognitive defusion (ability to recognize and label thoughts as "just thoughts" and let go of attachment or reaction to the thoughts themselves).
3. Learning to be present through use of mindfulness to observe pleasant and unpleasant experiences as they occur (eg, noticing feelings of comfort in bed).
4. Using self as context (one's ability to develop a broader awareness of their own core self) to have nonjudgmental stance toward sleep-related experiences and realize you are greater than your insomnia.
5. Clarify values that improve their QoL and focus attention away from sleep.
6. Establish committed action to behaviors in line with one's goals that favor pursuit of values despite experience of insomnia.

In ACT-based interventions for insomnia, the above elements are incorporated into treatment that also includes the behavioral components of insomnia treatment, such as sleep restriction and stimulus control. To demonstrate the differences between acceptance-based and ACT-based interventions to treat insomnia and CBT-I, **Table 1** outlines session by session treatment components of an ACT-based intervention titled Acceptance and the Behavioral Changes to treat Insomnia (ABC-I) created by Lavinia Fiorentino and Jennifer L. Martin,[24] compared with that of CBT-I.

To further illustrate the adaptation of ACT as a treatment modality for insomnia, **Table 2** illustrates examples of metaphors used to exemplify ACT concepts of acceptance and willingness, present moment focus and mindfulness, cognitive defusion, as well as traditional behavioral components (eg, sleep restriction).[24,25]

Mechanisms for Change: Cognitive Behavioral Therapy for Insomnia versus Acceptance and Commitment Therapy to Treat Primary Insomnia

There are several proposed mechanisms by which ACT-based interventions may be effective for the treatment of insomnia. Through the use of experiential acceptance and willingness, mindfulness and cognitive defusion, and values identification and committed action, individuals experiencing insomnia can increase flexibility, openness, and acceptance of a wide range of cognitive and emotional phenomena associated with sleep difficulties, as well as challenging insomnia-specific behavioral treatment components.

Generally, psychological inflexibility has been shown to be a significant predictor of insomnia severity and increased avoidance behaviors that are linked to sleep disturbances.[26,27] Therefore, borrowing components of acceptance and willingness from ACT may be beneficial to individuals with insomnia because it fosters experiential openness and flexibility, rather than suppression of difficult internal experiences or overregulation of psycho-physiological processes associated with sleep. It is theorized that disengagement from daily concerns involves letting go of controlled information processing by reducing verbal regulation and control, and increasing acceptance of spontaneously occurring physiological and mental processes (eg, sleep imagery). Acceptance may help to promote cognitive deactivation and physiological dearousal during initial sleep onset.[20]

Acceptance has also been shown to decrease counterproductive sleep effort, or what has been called the "attention effort syndrome," defined as the tendency of individuals with insomnia to struggle to control their sleep by "trying hard" to fall asleep (Espie and colleagues, 2006). This effortful attempt to sleep often results in a secondary arousal state, which contributes to increases in frustration and anxiety that fuels a vicious cycle of worsening the problem.[21,22,28] ACT may help individuals to decrease secondary distress by fostering acceptance and willingness to let go of the effort to fall asleep, thus decreasing this struggle over time.[20,22,29] Experiential acceptance and willingness may also be particularly beneficial in helping individuals with insomnia realize and internalize that sleep is not under voluntary control and fluctuations in sleep due to stressful events or other daily concerns are to be occasionally expected as part of the human experience.[20]

Furthermore, ACT may be helpful in supporting individuals with insomnia through difficult behavioral components of treatment, namely sleep restriction and stimulus control. Many individuals with insomnia struggle with anxiety and fears about losing sleep, being fatigued during the day, or maintaining a particular amount of sleep. An acceptance-based approach can help to increase adherence to sleep restriction and other difficult behavioral components of insomnia treatment (eg, the stimulus control recommendation to get out of bed when struggling with sleep during the night) by facilitating a willingness to experience short-term discomfort associated with behavioral recommendations for long-term

Table 1
Sample session outline: acceptance and the behavioral changes to treat insomnia, an acceptance and commitment therapy-based insomnia treatment, compared with cognitive behavioral therapy for insomnia

Session Number	ABC-I	CBT-I
Session 1 (postinitial evaluation):	• Introduce stimulus control and sleep hygiene • Identify values to foster acceptance of discomfort related to insomnia • Introduce mindfulness	• Goal setting and sleep education (2 process model; 3 Ps) • Rationale for sleep restriction • Introduce sleep restriction and stimulus control
Session 2:	• Sleep education (2 process model; 3 Ps model of insomnia) • Rational for sleep restriction • Introduce sleep restriction • Mindfulness practice	• Introduce sleep hygiene • Maintenance of sleep restriction
Session 3:	• Introduce cognitive defusion and self as context • Mindfulness practice • Maintenance of sleep restriction	• Introduce cognitive therapy, including identifying and challenging thoughts related to sleep • Maintenance of sleep restriction and continued practice of stimulus control guidelines
Session 4:	• Review of cognitive defusion, self as context • Maintenance of sleep restriction • Mindfulness practice	• Maintenance of sleep restriction, stimulus control, and cognitive training
Sessions 5–8:	• Review • Maintenance of sleep restriction • Mindfulness practice • Relapse prevention	• Introduce relaxation training • Maintenance of sleep restriction, stimulus control, cognitive therapy • Relapse prevention overview

benefit, particularly when those benefits are linked to the individuals' life values.[22]

Further, cognitive defusion and mindfulness components of ACT may help individuals manage the cognitive components of insomnia. Individuals with insomnia tend to have a larger number of negative thoughts at night and may use more thought-control strategies (thought suppression, reappraisal, and worrying) than healthy sleepers. They may also struggle more with thought suppression and hold fairly rigid beliefs about their sleep.[30–33] These thought-control strategies require effort and contribute to longer sleep latencies and worse sleep quality.[34] The experiential avoidance that individuals use in an attempt to control their cognitive and psychological experiences (eg, thought control) can maintain their insomnia.[20] Furthermore, a focus on changing thoughts or experiences related to insomnia (eg, frustration associated with sleep latency) can sometimes lead to additional attempts to overcontrol these thoughts at a time when increased cognitive mentation is counter to the ultimate goal of achieving sleep initiation. As traditional CBT-I teaches individuals cognitive restructuring of unpleasant thoughts or dysfunctional beliefs, ACT proposes that individuals can decrease the struggle with these inner experiences by letting go of the attempt to change them. By engaging in present moment focus and cognitive defusion strategies, individuals can use mindfulness to notice thoughts that originate while trying to fall asleep without judgement or need to alter the thought. Cognitive defusion further allows individuals to shift their relation with the content of their thoughts.[21] **Fig. 2** shows the use of ACT-based cognitive defusion strategies versus traditional cognitive therapy (eg, thought restructuring) to manage a sleep-related thought.

Finally, a focus on individual values to increase motivation and adherence to eventually achieve long-term sleep outcomes is a key component of ACT for insomnia. It is common among individuals with insomnia to place an exaggerated value on sleep and subsequent tiredness and fatigue resulting from lack of sleep or poor sleep quality.

Table 2
Sleep-related metaphors that can be incorporated into treatment of insomnia to address challenges

Learning how to surf	Getting good sleep is a lot like learning how to surf. What do you need to go surfing? A surf board? A wet suit? Sunscreen? Checking the weather report? Going down to the water? Paddling out? And then what? You wait for the waves. There is nothing you can do to make the waves comes faster or stronger. You wait for whatever wave you get that day. That is our parallel to sleep: There is a lot that we are going to do to make the conditions are right for sleep and help you learn how to ride the sleep waves. However, on any one night, there is not a lot that you or I can do to make a sleep wave come any faster or stronger. You must accept the sleep waves that you get and trust that you will become a better sleep surfer in time *Purpose*: Designed to convey two aspects of fostering good sleep: (1) Preparation for a good night's sleep (sleep hygiene rules) such as when as a surfer prepares to have a good surfing experience by waking up early, waxing their board, wearing a wet suit, stretchlng, and so forth and (2) Giving up control over sleep by using mindfulness and an accepting stance that sleep will come (such as a surfer waits for a wave to arrive)
Finger trap	*Give patient finger trap and ask them to put their fingers inside Have you ever played with one of these before? What happens when you try to pull your fingers apart? The more that you struggle to release your fingers, the tighter the trap becomes and the more difficult it becomes to free yourself. The trick is to do the opposite of what you think you should do: pushing your fingers together will loosen the trap and allow you to remove your fingers. Similarly to this trap, the more we struggle with our sleep, the more elusive sleep becomes. Instead, we will be trying some strategies that at first might seem counterinitiative to what you think will work in order to promote better sleep. Instead of struggling to sleep, we must relax and let sleep unfold naturally. *Purpose*: A reminder to "stop trying to sleep." The woven bamboo tubes (finger traps) illustrate the effectiveness of what may seem counterintuitive at times. In regards to sleep, individuals learn that what they may think is counterintuitive (eg, stop trying to fall asleep, sleep restriction) may actually promote sleep
Leaves on a stream	"Leaves on a stream meditation"[24] involves asking individuals to attend to their breath and envision a stream. As thoughts and emotions come up during mindfulness exercise, guide individuals in putting each thought on a leaf and watching it float down the stream. *Purpose*: A classic ACT meditation that incorporates breath work, focusing on the physical body and senses, and a visualization depicting one's thoughts as flowing downward leaves on a stream. This exercise promotes practice of mindfulness and cognitive defusion (if you can imagine your thoughts as leaves on a stream, you cannot be your thoughts)
Pizza dough/silly putty	Have you ever made pizza from pizza dough? What happens when the dough is rolled out too far? The dough become thin and breaks. When this happens, we are unable to add more dough to the holes. Instead, we must ball up the dough and start over again. This is the approach we are going to take with your sleep. You have cast a wide net for sleep, hoping that you will get more sleep as a result. Unfortunately, you have holes in your sleep. Similar to the dough, we are going to ball up your sleep to an amount of time your body is currently capable of producing (which we will know from your sleep diary). Once we eliminate the holes in your sleep (ie, you start sleeping more solidly), we will start to roll out your sleep (ie, increase your time in bed). *Purpose*: Used to describe the concept of sleep restriction therapy and how our sleep quality and quantity is improved over time. The metaphor uses pizza dough or silly putty to explain that we first work on consolidating sleep and then work on expanding sleep again once we increase the quality of it, as if we were rolling the dough out again

Cleaning out your closet/renovating your home	When was the last time you cleaned out your closet? Usually one of the first steps is taking everything out to sort through it before you put it back in. This often means that the mess looks much bigger before it begins to look organized. This is a similar process to the work we are doing. Some aspects of your sleep (eg, fatigue, mood) might get worse before they get better as your body is working through these changes. However, like cleaning out your closet, the mess is still on the road to a cleaner closet! *Purpose*: In behavioral treatment of insomnia, symptoms (eg, fatigue, sleepiness, mood) often get worse before they get better. These metaphors help individuals compare this process to other difficult activities, such as cleaning out your closet or renovating your home
Physicalizing visualization	Another thing you might do when you encounter feelings and thoughts about your insomnia is to externalize these experiences outside of your body. If these experiences were outside of your body, what shape would they have? If you could put these thoughts and feelings outside your body, what color would they be? How big would they be? Would they be rough or smooth, silky or like granite? What would they sound or smell like? *Purpose*: In this experiential exercise, the therapist guides the patient in visualizing their insomnia, as well as their feelings and thoughts about insomnia. By visualizing these experiences as objects outside of their body, individuals are able to feel like they are more than these experiences and are not fused to them
Clean versus dirty discomfort	There are many ways that I can respond to pain and discomfort. Let us say I stub my toe. I might initially feel the pain and then take steps to manage and soothe the pain (eg, put ice on my foot). We call this clean discomfort. Instead, I might respond by telling myself "I'm so clumsy." We call this dirty discomfort; when I add negative self-judgements to my experience of pain, which ultimately makes my experience of pain worse. We cannot escape experiencing pain and discomfort but we can change how we approach these experiences and how we treat ourselves when we do feel pain. *Purpose*: These concepts refer to the difference between experiencing pain or discomfort versus applying negative judgement to the experience of pain. The overall discomfort and pain is exacerbated when adding dirty pain/discomfort versus clean pain/discomfort alone. This metaphor can help individuals recognize self-judgement and take a self-compassionate approach instead of criticism
Take your mind for a walk	This is an experiential exercise in which the provider and patient go for a walk (or imagine doing so). The provider walks slightly behind the patient, talking directly into the patient's ear pretending to be their mind. The provider offers a variety of comments (positive, critical, and neutral) to emulate the patient's self-judgements (personalizing to the patient's common self-talk statements). The patient's role is to "listen to their mind" and notice resulting feeling and actions. The patient should be made aware that no comment "literally" stopped the patient from moving forward *Purpose*: The aim of this exercise is to allow the patient the opportunity to notice the variety of things their mind is saying at any given time, some thoughts helpful while others are harmful. The patient may come to understand that they have the choice of how to act and relate toward their own mental chatter and are encouraged to act according to their values, regardless of what thoughts their minds give them
Two plates scale	Present a picture of a two-plated scale and explain that their insomnia is on one of the plates and their willingness to accept their experience of insomnia is on the other. Demonstrate what happens to the scale with individuals who are unwilling to accept their experience (ie, the insomnia rises). Demonstrate again that if they experience more willingness to accept their experience of insomnia, the insomnia plate becomes more balanced or even lighter than the willingness plate *Purpose*: Used to describe the relationship between willingness, acceptance, and suffering. This metaphor can further illustrate the concept of clean and dirty discomfort

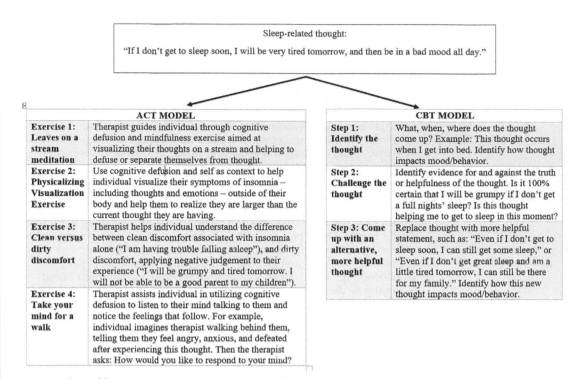

Fig. 2. Outline of how Acceptance and Commitment Therapy (ACT) and Cognitive Behavioral Therapy (CBT) approaches can be used to address sleep-focused thoughts".

Consequentially, individuals with chronic insomnia may lose sight of some of their life values because their attention is directed toward control of their sleepiness or fatigue.[21,22] Individuals may make concessions in nonsleep-related values in the service of symptom management. Thus, value-based goal setting and committed action may increase willingness to adhere to difficult behavioral recommendations in the service of nonsleep-related values (eg, getting out of bed at the same time every day to exercise instead of sleeping in after getting a poor night's sleep due to a value of health and wellness). Individuals are encouraged to commit to actions related to their values, such as engaging in activities instead of canceling them due to symptoms on insomnia, and to use cognitive defusion and acceptance of thoughts and feelings that may promote avoidance of these activities. The emphasis on value-based living at the onset and throughout insomnia treatment may help individuals to see beyond the discomfort of both insomnia symptoms and the challenging treatment components, and engage fully in treatment that is in the service of their values.

Research Outcomes

Although nascent, studies examining outcomes of acceptance-based interventions for insomnia demonstrate decreases in sleep disturbance as well as improvements in QoL. It is notable that most studies to date have examined the effectiveness of ACT-only interventions: not including insomnia-specific behavioral interventions such as sleep restriction and stimulus control. In a pilot study examining the effectiveness of ACT-only (not including insomnia-specific behavioral interventions) in nonresponders to CBT-I, ACT improved sleep-related QoL and subjective sleep quality despite the absence of substantive changes in total sleep time.[29] A systematic review of intervention studies conducted by Salari and colleagues (2020) showed that ACT has a significant effect on insomnia, termed primary insomnia by authors indicating insomnia not caused by comorbid conditions, and sleep quality. Specifically, the review included 19 intervention studies, 3 of which have examined the effect of ACT interventions on primary insomnia. Of those studies, ACT-only interventions were associated with improvements in insomnia, including sleep duration (total sleep time), subjective sleep quality, and sleep-related cognitive and emotional processes.[35–37] It was also suggested that improvements in symptoms can occur even within the first few weeks of treatment.[36,37] Moreover, these studies found significant decreases in experiential avoidance, dysfunctional beliefs and attitudes about sleep, difficulties in emotional regulation, and severity of depressive symptoms, as well as sleep acceptance improvements over time in the ACT group when compared with the active control group.[35,37] This suggests the theoretical underpinnings of ACT were important to symptom improvement. The remainder of the studies included in this review indicated that ACT had a significant impact on comorbid insomnia, or insomnia occurring with other diseases, such as chronic pain, cancer, or fibromyalgia.

Results of 2 small studies using the ACT-based intervention titled ABC-I demonstrate clinically meaningful improvements in sleep outcome measures for participants who underwent the ABC-I intervention. Of note, the ABC-I intervention includes both components of ACT and insomnia-specific behavioral components.[24] Across both ABC-I pilot studies, researchers found improvements in insomnia severity and reduced sleep effort at posttreatment. Furthermore, one of the pilot studies also showed reduced self-reported sleep disruptions, increased in sleep quality, and no attrition (eg, all participants enrolled in ABC-I completed treatment, even those who has previously dropped out of CBT-I). Existing literature suggest promising results for the use of ACT to treat insomnia either as a standalone treatment or in conjunction with insomnia-specific behavioral interventions.

Use of Acceptance and Commitment Therapy in subpopulations of individuals with insomnia

Although CBT-I is highly effective for individuals with comorbid medical and mental health conditions, these conditions sometimes present specific challenges to treatment. This section outlines the theoretical rationale for using ACT-based exercises in these circumstances. For example, individuals who have experienced trauma at night may hold the thought, "Sleep is not safe because bad things happen at night." The cognitive therapy approach of challenging and restructuring this thought may be effective for some individuals, although others may think it invalidates their traumatic experiences. However, using an ACT approach, the individual would not need to change this initial thought but rather relate to it in a way that places less emphasis on the thought itself and validates the rationale for the thought to occur. One could work with the patient to acknowledge this meaningful thought while still taking steps toward better sleep so they can live a life consistent with what they value most (eg, being active during the day with their family).

This approach can also be useful with older adults who suffer from multiple chronic conditions and those suffering from chronic pain that affects sleep. In some instances, a patient may not be able to achieve "ideal" sleep or to sleep as well as they did earlier in life. Using an ACT-based approach, one can explore these issues through experiential exercises that highlight differences between actual "pain" and psychological "suffering." This approach can help individuals to create realistic expectations and reduce counterproductive sleep effort.

The idea that thoughts can be helpful versus unhelpful and that they can or should be changed is also a notion that is not shared by all individuals in all cultures. Some individuals may find this notion inconsistent with their own personal values or belief system, and therefore may not believe that their provider truly understands their symptoms and experiences. The adaptability of ACT across cultural and diversity factors has been previously discussed as an important area of study.[38] Since the center of the approach is the patient's own values and lived experiences and not the therapist's assessment of whether a thought is helpful or unhelpful, ACT may therefore be appropriate for individuals from a variety of cultural backgrounds.

SUMMARY

In contrast to CBT-I, ACT proposes that the process of attempting to control, reduce or eliminate thoughts, emotions or physical sensations associated with sleep contributes to greater struggle with sleep difficulties, thus leading to increased symptomology and suffering. The goal of acceptance-based and ACT-based interventions is to assist individuals in managing insomnia symptoms by using acceptance and willingness, cognitive defusion and mindfulness, self as context, and values as a means to commit to implementing changes that will improve sleep. Differences exist in the structure of acceptance-based and ACT-based insomnia interventions in the literature, with some including typical behavioral components of CBT-I, and some using acceptance strategies alone. Overall, research examining outcomes of acceptance-based interventions for insomnia demonstrate improvements in both sleep outcomes and QoL. Furthermore, ACT interventions can be uniquely tailored to specific values that individuals identify at the outset of treatment, particularly those values affected by insomnia. An ACT approach may be useful for individuals with comorbid mental health and medical conditions to focus on meaningful changes in sleep behaviors that bring them closer to valued living, as well as facilitate adaptation of insomnia treatment to be patient-centered and account for lived experiences that may differ by sociocultural background.

CLINICS CARE POINTS

- Acceptance and commitment therapy (ACT) is a third wave behavioral therapy that can be used as an alternative or adjunctive approach in the treatment of insomnia.

- ACT-based interventions for insomnia can be used to increase psychological and behavioral flexibility regarding sleep and sleep difficulties.

- ACT tools such as experiential acceptance and willingness, mindfulness and cognitive defusion, and values identification and committed action may assist individuals experiencing insomnia to increase openness and acceptance through: 1) targeting avoidance behaviors and control strategies; 2) counterproductive sleep effort; 3) tolerance of short-term discomfort; 4) and value-based living.

- Acceptance and ACT-based interventions have been shown to result in significant improvements in sleep outcomes, such as reductions in insomnia severity and sleep effort, well as improvement in sleep-related quality of life and subjective sleep quality.

- ACT-based approaches to insomnia treatment may improve patient-centered care due to broad adaptability of ACT across diverse lived experiences.

DISCLOSURE

This study was supported by VA HSR&D IIR 16-244. Dr. Martin was supported by VA HSR&D RCS 20-191 and NIH/NHLBI K24 HL143055. This study was also supported by VA Greater Los Angeles Healthcare System (VAGLAHS) Geriatric Research, Education and Clinical Center (GRECC), VA Office of Academic Affiliations (Saldana), and VA Greater Los Angeles Healthcare System Mental Health Service (McGowan).

REFERENCES

1. Edinger JD, Means MK, Carney CE, et al. Psychomotor performance defcits and their relation to prior nights' sleep among individuals with primary insomnia. Sleep 2008;31(5):599–607.
2. Walker MP, Stickgold R. Sleep-dependent learning and memory consolidation. Neuron 2004;44(1):121–33.
3. Kessler RC, Berglund PA, Coulouvrat C, et al. Insomnia and the performance of US workers: results from the America insomnia survey. Sleep 2011;34(9):1161–71.
4. Zammit GK, Weiner J, Damato N, et al. Quality of life in people with insomnia. Sleep 1999;22(Suppl 2):S379–85.
5. Ohayon MM. Relationship between chronic painful physical condition and insomnia. J Psychiatr Res 2005;39(2):151–9.
6. Taylor DJ, Lichstein KL, Durrence HH, et al. Epidemiology of insomnia, depression, and anxiety. Sleep 2005;28(11):1457–64.
7. Qaseem A, Kansagara D, Forciea M, et al. Clinical guidelines committee of the american college of P. management of chronic insomnia disorder in adults: a clinical practice guideline from the american college of physicians. Ann Intern Med 2016;165(2):125–33.
8. Edinger JD, Arnedt JT, Bertisch SM, et al. Behavioral and psychological treatments for chronic insomnia disorder in adults: an American Academy of Sleep Medicine systematic review, meta-analysis, and GRADE assessment. J Clin Sleep Med 2021;17(2):263–98.
9. Irwin MR, Cole JC, Nicassio PM. Comparative meta-analysis of behavioral interventions for insomnia and their efficacy in middle-aged adults and in older adults 55+ years of age. Health Psychol 2006;25(1):3.
10. Cunningham JE, Shapiro CM. Cognitive Behavioural Therapy for Insomnia (CBT-I) to treat depression: a systematic review. J psychosomatic Res 2018;106:1–12.
11. Talbot LS, Maguen S, Metzler TJ, et al. Cognitive behavioral therapy for insomnia in posttraumatic stress disorder: a randomized controlled trial. Sleep 2014;37(2):327–41.
12. Vitiello MV, Rybarczyk B, Von Korff M, et al. Cognitive behavioral therapy for insomnia improves sleep and decreases pain in older adults with co-morbid insomnia and osteoarthritis. J Clin Sleep Med 2009;5(4):355–62.
13. Fung CH, Martin JL, Josephson K, et al. Efficacy of cognitive behavioral therapy for insomnia in older adults with occult sleep-disordered breathing. Psychosom Med 2016;78(5):629.
14. Perlis ML, Smith MT, Orff H, et al. The effects of modafinil and cognitive behavior therapy on sleep continuity in patients with primary insomnia. Sleep 2004;27(4):715–25.
15. Hayes SC. Acceptance and commitment therapy, relational frame theory, and the third wave of behavioral and cognitive therapies. Behav Ther 2004;35(4):639–65.
16. Hayes SC, Strosahl KD, Wilson KG. Acceptance and commitment therapy: the process and practice of

mindful change. New York, London: Guilford Press; 2011.

17. Hayes SC, Pistorello J, Levin ME. Acceptance and commitment therapy as a unified model of behavior change. Couns Psychol 2012;40(7): 976–1002.

18. Gloster AT, Walder N, Levin ME, et al. The empirical status of acceptance and commitment therapy: a review of meta-analyses. J Contextual Behav Sci 2020; 18:181–92.

19. Powers MB, Vörding MBZVS, Emmelkamp PM. Acceptance and commitment therapy: a meta-analytic review. Psychother Psychosom 2009;78(2): 73–80.

20. Lundh L-G. The role of acceptance and mindfulness in the treatment of insomnia. J Cogn Psychother 2005;19(1):29–39.

21. Ong JC, Ulmer CS, Manber R. Improving sleep with mindfulness and acceptance: a metacognitive model of insomnia. Behav Res Ther 2012;50(11): 651–60.

22. Dalrymple KL, Fiorentino L, Politi MC, et al. Incorporating principles from acceptance and commitment therapy into cognitive-behavioral therapy for insomnia: a case example. J Contemp Psychotherapy 2010;40(4):209–17.

23. deok Baik K. (2015). Evaluating acceptance and commitment therapy for insomnia: a randomized controlled trial (Publication No. 3726703) [Doctoral Disseration, Bowling Green State University]. ProQuest Disserations & Theses Global.

24. Fiorentino L, Martin JL, Alessi CA. The ABCs of Insomnia (ABC-I): An Acceptance Commitment Therapy (ACT)-Based Insomnia Treatment Development Study: Pilot Results and Future Directions. In: Sedky K, Nazir R, Bennett D, editors. Sleep Medicine and Mental Health: A Guide for Psychiatrists and Other Healthcare Professionals. 1st Edition. Switzerland: Springer Nature; 2020.

25. Harris R. Act made simple: an easy-to-read primer on acceptance and commitment. Oakland, California, United States: New Harbinger; 2009.

26. Hall M, Thayer JF, Germain A, et al. Psychological stress is associated with heightened physiological arousal during NREM sleep in primary insomnia. Behav Sleep Med 2007;5(3):178–93.

27. McCracken LM, Williams JL, Tang NK. Psychological flexibility may reduce insomnia in persons with chronic pain: a preliminary retrospective study. Pain Med 2011;12(6):904–12.

28. Espie CA, Broomfield NM, MacMahon KM, et al. The attention–intention–effort pathway in the development of psychophysiologic insomnia: a theoretical review. Sleep Med Rev 2006;10(4):215–45.

29. Hertenstein E, Thiel N, Lüking M, et al. Quality of life improvements after acceptance and commitment therapy in nonresponders to cognitive behavioral therapy for primary insomnia. Psychotherapy and psychosomatics 2014;83(6):371–3.

30. Harvey AG. I can't sleep, my mind is racing! an investigation of strategies of thought control in insomnia Allison G. Harvey. Behav Cogn Psychotherapy 2001;29(1):3–11.

31. Harvey AG. The attempted suppression of presleep cognitive activity in insomnia. Cogn Ther Res 2003; 27(6):593–602.

32. Morin CM. Insomnia: psychological assessment and management. New York: Guilford press; 1993.

33. Watts FN, Coyle K, East MP. The contribution of worry to insomnia. Br J Clin Psychol 1994;33(2):211–20.

34. Thomsen DK, Mehlsen MY, Christensen S, et al. Rumination—relationship with negative mood and sleep quality. Pers Individ Dif 2003;34(7):1293–301.

35. Lappalainen P, Langrial S, Oinas-Kukkonen H, et al. ACT for sleep-internet-delivered self-help ACT for sub-clinical and clinical insomnia: a randomized controlled trial. J Contextual Behav Sci 2019;12: 119–27.

36. Zakiei A, Khazaie H. The effectiveness of acceptance and commitment therapy on insomnia patients (A single-arm trial plan). J Turkish Sleep Medicine-Turk Uyku Tibbi Dergisi 2019;6(3):65–73.

37. Zakiei A, Khazaie H, Rostampour M, et al. Acceptance and Commitment Therapy (ACT) improves sleep quality, experiential avoidance, and emotion regulation in individuals with insomnia—results from a randomized interventional study. Life 2021; 11(2):133.

38. Woidneck MR, Pratt KM, Gundy JM, et al. Exploring cultural competence in acceptance and commitment therapy outcomes. Prof Psychol Res Pr 2012; 43(3):227.

Biofeedback as an Adjunct or Alternative Intervention to Cognitive Behavioral Therapy for Insomnia

Stephanie Kremer, PsyD[a],*, Tanecia Blue, PhD, ABPP[b]

KEYWORDS

- Biofeedback • Insomnia • Neurofeedback • Comorbid
- Cognitive behavioral therapy for insomnia (CBT-I) • Adjunctive • Alternative intervention

KEY POINTS

- Biofeedback is an effective intervention that uses training in self-regulation through a variety of modalities to ameliorate symptoms and/or improve performance.
- Biofeedback has demonstrated efficacy in the treatment in a range of disorders, including insomnia.
- CBT-I has limitations that may be addressed with biofeedback as an adjunct intervention or, if necessary, an alternative in combination with other treatments (e.g., sleep hygiene).
- Methodological concerns and mixed results in research on biofeedback for insomnia necessitate future well-designed studies to establish its clinical effectiveness in insomnia treatment.

INTRODUCTION

Biofeedback training is the process of learning self-regulation for the purpose of improving health and ameliorating symptoms.[1] Various forms of biofeedback training, alone or in combination with other treatments, have shown to be effective interventions in the treatment of a range of psychiatric and chronic health disorders.[1,2] Biofeedback involves the use of physiologic measurements that allow an individual to make changes to physiology to learn to improve health and performance. Information about physiologic functions, such as heart rate, muscle activity, breathing, and brain waves, is obtained through the use of instruments and provided to the individual in real time to allow changes to be made to achieve a certain criterion in that domain. Ideally, these changes are maintained over time without the use of an instrument.[3]

Insomnia disorder is the complaint regarding *dissatisfaction* with sleep quality or quantity associated with difficulty initiating or maintaining sleep or early morning awakenings occurring 3 or more nights per week with a minimum duration of 3 months when opportunity for sleep was available. This disturbance results in significant impairment in daytime functioning and/or clinically significant distress and is not due to the effects of a substance or better explained by a coexisting disorder.[4] About 6% to 10% of adults with symptoms of insomnia meet the full diagnostic criteria.[4] Moreover, one-third of adults report some symptoms of insomnia, with symptoms increasing with age.[5] Some studies indicate the rate of adults

[a] Department of Psychiatry and Biobehavioral Sciences, UCLA David Geffen School of Medicine, UCLA Insomnia Clinic, Cousins Center for Psychoneuroimmunology, 300 Medical Plaza, Suite 3200A, Los Angeles, CA 90095, USA; [b] VA Pacific Islands Healthcare System, 459 Patterson Road, Honolulu, HI 96819, USA
* Corresponding author.
E-mail address: skremer@mednet.ucla.edu

Sleep Med Clin 18 (2023) 85–93
https://doi.org/10.1016/j.jsmc.2022.10.003
1556-407X/23/© 2022 Elsevier Inc. All rights reserved.

reporting insomnia symptoms could be as high as 50%.[5–7] Chronic insomnia is more common among women and those from lower socioeconomic status (SES) groups.[5–7] Although sleep difficulties are highly prevalent in communities of color and lower SES groups, they are poorly recognized and underdiagnosed[8]; thus, accurate rates are difficult to determine.

Insomnia is frequently comorbid with other medical or psychiatric disorders.[4] Primary and secondary subtypes of insomnia are no longer used by the Diagnostic and Statistical Manual-Fifth Edition or the International Classification of Sleep Disorders-Third Edition ,given the overlap in symptoms and frequency of comorbid diagnoses making a causal relationship difficult to determine.[9]

During the Covid-19 pandemic, there has been a significant increase in reported symptoms of insomnia, depression, anxiety, posttraumatic stress disorder, and psychological distress in the general adult population.[10–12] A systematic review and meta-analysis by Jahrami and colleagues looking at 13 different countries indicated that patients with COVID-19 seemed to be the most affected by sleep problems with a pooled rate of almost 75%.[13] Others have also raised the concern for increased rates of insomnia in health-care workers,[10] patients with noninfectious chronic disease, and people in quarantine.[11]

Given the high rates of reported sleep difficulty and insomnia, as well as the associated adverse health consequences[14] and high costs,[15] there is a need for safe, effective treatments to address ever growing sleep problems. Psychological and behavioral treatments have consistently proven to be effective and widely accepted treatments of insomnia.[9,16] These treatments also help reduce or avoid the adverse consequences of pharmacotherapy.[17] Cognitive behavioral therapy for insomnia (CBT-I) has generally been considered the standard and first-line treatment of insomnia as recommended by the American College of Physicians and the recent task force for the American Academy of Sleep Medicine.[9,17] CBT-I has also proven efficacious in the treatment of insomnia comorbid with or occurring in the context of medical or psychiatric disorders.[18,19]

Although CBT-I is an effective and safe intervention, some patients may not be appropriate candidates. Additionally, approximately 20% of CBT-I patients are considered nonresponders.[20] Cho and colleagues discussed patient-related attributes that predict greater adherence, and consequently, benefit from CBT-I.[21] For example, it was noted that those with a shorter sleep duration (ie, <6 hours) or with inadequately treated psychiatric comorbidities may have a less favorable response to CBT-I. Additionally, shorter sleep duration may complicate the implementation of a core component of CBT-I treatment, sleep restriction. Individuals may be hesitant to engage in cognitive behavioral treatment due to the stigma sometimes associated with psychotherapy or mental health disorders. Others may be reluctant to engage in or adhere to the behavior change required to implement the core components of CBT-I, sleep/time in bed restriction, and stimulus control (eg, limiting time in bed to only sleep and intimacy, getting out of bed when not sleeping). There are other instances when CBT-I may be contraindicated or should be used with a high level of caution, for example, in the presence of seizure or bipolar disorders.[22]

Biofeedback for Insomnia

Biofeedback is frequently referenced in the literature and used in clinical practice as an intervention for insomnia. It is similar to CBT-I in that both are active interventions that require participant engagement and adherence for desired results. Biofeedback is considered safe with generally few cautions in its application, which can typically be addressed by a skilled provider.[23] Biofeedback offers a promising alternative or adjunctive intervention when CBT-I is either inadequate or may be contraindicated, or for those who are reluctant to engage in traditional psychotherapy or pharmacotherapy. An approach using biofeedback may also be an attractive option for those seeking a more tangible mind–body approach with immediate physiologic data for reinforcement and motivation.

History and Rationale

Early interest in biofeedback for insomnia was driven by the hypothesized relationship between physiologic arousal and insomnia.[24] Early psychophysiological interventions for insomnia focused on reduction of muscle tension using electromyography (EMG) and included comparing various forms of relaxation training.[25,26] The results of these early studies were mixed, and EMG biofeedback eventually declined in popularity as a treatment of insomnia.[27]

Neurofeedback, a type of biofeedback that involves using operant conditioning techniques to train brain waves, has demonstrated beneficial effects on insomnia.[28–30] These interventions are designed to target the cognitive, somatic, and cortical hyperarousal that is believed to be characteristic of insomnia and are associated with improvements in perceived insomnia severity, quality of life, and daytime functioning.[31] Early neurofeedback studies described the relation between the role of sleep spindle production and insomnia. Sensorimotor rhythm (SMR) neurofeedback is a type of neurofeedback identified as having an impact on sleep and is currently recognized as one of the standard neurofeedback protocols.[32] Subsequent neurofeedback studies have identified different protocols that target training other brain waves (eg, theta/beta to promote sleep initiation); however, SMR neurofeedback is the most significantly studied for insomnia during the longest period of time.[20]

Heart rate variability biofeedback (HRV-BF) is a relatively newer biofeedback modality used in the treatment of insomnia.[33] HRV-BF is an intervention intended to train the oscillations of the heartbeat to match breathing with heart rate patterns. The changes in the autonomic nervous system (ANS) affect a wide range of bodily functions and disorders, including insomnia. HRV-BF can restore dysfunctional autonomic responses and most importantly improve parasympathetic tone. Thus, HRV biofeedback can target the hyperexcitability of the sympathetic nervous system associated with insomnia.[34] Resonant frequency breathing, which is taught during this type of biofeedback training, is associated with improved sleep quality and improvements in daytime impairments.[34,35]

Current Evidence

Two 2019 systematic reviews on the use of biofeedback in the treatment of insomnia indicated mixed results and overall limitations in the research due to study design and quality (eg, small sample sizes, lack of control group).[31,36] Overall, they concluded that some results may be promising but more research with improved design was needed to determine benefits. Similarly, a 2021 nonsystematic review of neurofeedback in the treatment of insomnia also noted methodological barriers but indicated the studies are encouraging.[37] A recent pilot RCT by Kwan and colleagues demonstrated that a neurofeedback protocol was comparable in efficacy to CBT-I.[38] Other recent studies demonstrate the promise of biofeedback in the treatment of insomnia comorbid with other disorders.[39,40]

Biofeedback for Disorders Comorbid with Insomnia

Spielman's 3P model describes the process by which insomnia becomes chronic.[41] The model suggests that insomnia is initiated through the interaction of predisposing (eg, family history of sleep difficulties, medical disorder) and precipitating factors (eg, acute illness, recent stressor).

Compensatory behaviors, termed perpetuating factors, later increase the mismatch between sleep opportunity and sleep ability. CBT-I targets perpetuating factors such as engaging in nonsleep behaviors in bed and spending increased amounts of time in bed trying to sleep. Biofeedback may be most useful in addressing the precipitating factors such as stress and acute or chronic health disorders.

Given that symptoms of insomnia are comorbid with most disorders,[42] a stepped care approach that allows for multifaceted interventions aimed at symptoms of both insomnia and comorbid disorders may be the most advantageous route.[43] Biofeedback has been used successfully in the treatment of many disorders frequently comorbid with insomnia.[20,39,44,45] Comorbidities with insomnia seem to be bidirectional.[43] Biofeedback used as an adjunct to CBT-I in the treatment of comorbidities may address comorbidities, as well as hasten sleep gains.[43] A 2021 systematic review of HRV-BF including 9 RCTs indicated significant improvements in stress-related disorders, such as post-traumatic stress disorder (PTSD), panic disorder, and depression, with evidence of more significant improvements when combined with CBT or treatment as usual.[1] Another 2021 systematic review on HRV-BF and chronic disease management found that HRV-BF could be an effective component in the treatment of multiple chronic health conditions, such as cardiovascular disease, hypertension, asthma, anxiety, depression, and sleep disturbance.[2] Of the studies in this review assessing sleep disturbance specifically, improvements in sleep quality were shown in anxiety disorders, major depressive disorder, and PTSD.

Cardiovascular Disease

Sleep disturbance is highly comorbid with many cardiovascular diseases. Additionally, sleep duration is a risk factor for developing coronary heart disease, diabetes mellitus, and hypertension.[46] HRV-BF training improves ANS functioning and is associated with improvements in various cardiovascular diseases and sleep.[2,47] Biofeedback is also efficacious in the treatment of hypertension.[47]

Psychological Disorders

Insomnia symptoms are present in most anxiety disorders.[48–51] Conversely, anxiety is a common symptom reported by those seeking treatment of insomnia and, similar to depression, may complicate treatment engagement and response. The cerebral cortex may link anxiety and sleep disturbance anatomically and neurobiologically.[52]

Evidence suggests those with anxiety disorders and poor sleep may have worse outcomes than those with an independent anxiety disorder.[49,50] Treating co-occurring insomnia may be critical to improved outcomes. Biofeedback has demonstrated efficacy in the treatment of anxiety disorders,[53–55] and reduced hyperarousal is associated with improved symptoms of both anxiety and insomnia.

Sleep disturbance is a hallmark of PTSD with as many as 90% of individuals with this disorder reporting symptoms of insomnia.[56,57] There is a bidirectional relationship between PTSD and sleep problems.[52] HRV-BF has demonstrated strong positive effects on the amelioration of PTSD symptoms to include associated sleep disturbance.[20] Neurofeedback also shows promising results in the reduction of severity of PTSD symptoms, including sleep disturbance.[58] In a recent RCT, PTSD and insomnia symptoms as measured by a symptom checklist were significantly improved in the neurofeedback group compared with the control.[40]

Insomnia symptoms may occur in 80% to more than 90% of the cases of clinical depression[59,60] and approximately 40% of people diagnosed with depression meet the diagnostic criteria for insomnia disorder.[61] In individuals with depression, baroreflex receptor sensitivity seems to be lower,[62] and there is evidence of lower HRV.[63] HRV-BF targets vagal nerve innervation. Training an individual to breathe at coherence stimulates a vagal baroreflex response, which results in feelings of relaxation and subjectively improved well-being. HRV-BF has demonstrated a moderate positive effect on symptoms of depression.[44] Improved sleep quality and presleep arousal, as well as improved symptoms of anxiety and depression, were demonstrated in a recent case-control study of HRV-BF in patients with major depressive disorder and comorbid insomnia symptoms[39]

Pain Disorders

Insomnia and chronic pain are comorbid in up to 80% of individuals with chronic pain.[64] The relationship between pain and sleep seems to be mediated by multiple neurobiological systems or pathways (eg, melatonin, HPA axis).[65] For example, evidence suggest that the HPA axis may mediate the relation between sleep disturbance and pain sensitivity.[65] Sleep disturbance can affect pain intensity, pain duration, and psychosocial functioning.[66] Biofeedback can address both sleep and pain. HRV-BF improves vagal tone, which has an impact on pain and insomnia.[67] A

recent review of several studies on chronic pain and fibromyalgia concluded that biofeedback, specifically HRV-BF, is related to decreased pain.[68]

Neurologic Disorders

There is a neurobiological association between attention-deficit/hyperactivity-disorder (ADHD) and short sleep duration. ADHD is particularly associated with sleep onset insomnia in a large subset of ADHD patients.[32] Neurofeedback is considered efficacious in the treatment of ADHD and may serve as a useful adjunct to CBT-I in patients with ADHD.[20,45] In those patients, treatment with SMR neurofeedback is hypothesized to normalize sleep and improve ADHD symptoms by training the sleep-spindle circuitry.[32]

Insomnia is common in epilepsy and is associated with poor seizure control.[69] Moreover, sleep deprivation lowers seizure threshold, which may contraindicate the use of sleep restriction in CBT-I with many patients who have epilepsy.[19] SMR neurofeedback is well-established as an efficacious treatment of epilepsy with promising evidence for improvements in sleep.[70]

Insomnia, cognitive deficits, emotional distress, personality disturbance, and headaches are common symptoms of traumatic brain injury (TBI). In fact, insomnia and other sleep disturbances are one of the most frequent post-TBI complaints.[71] Although CBT-I is an effective treatment of insomnia in patients diagnosed with TBI,[72] biofeedback is a useful adjunct to treat the wide range of symptoms accompanying TBI and can improve quality of life and lower medication burden.[73]

Considerations

Access to care

Biofeedback is similar to CBT-I in that access to care is limited. For both interventions, there is a scarcity of providers trained to accommodate the need for services. The availability of biofeedback may also be limited by reimbursement difficulties and the high cost of equipment and provider training.[74] Additionally, insomnia is underdiagnosed in communities of color and lower SES groups, which further decreases access to specialized sleep medicine care.

Updated methods for expanding options in biofeedback may increase accessibility. Less expensive and portable equipment options are becoming more available for office and home use. Some biofeedback therapies are easy to integrate into a treatment session addressing comorbid disorders or in combination with CBT-I.[75]

Table 1
Comparison of Biofeedback for insomnia and cognitive behavioral therapy for insomnia

	Biofeedback	CBT-I
Typical treatment targets	Precipitating factors, hyperarousal	Perpetuating factors, increased focus on cognitive factors
Number of sessions	10–20, optional follow-ups	6–8, optional follow-ups
Cautions/ contraindications	Generally safe; severe and uncontrolled psychiatric conditions; some cardiac conditions; modify for some dermatologic conditions	Generally safe; inadequately controlled psychiatric disorders; short sleep duration; seizure disorders; bipolar disorder; Nonrapid eye movement parasomnias; nocturnal panic attacks; some simultaneous trauma treatments
Access to care	Limited due to availability of trained providers and cost of equipment; may be integrated into other treatments	Limited due to availability of trained providers; may be integrated with other treatments
Telehealth	Yes, with specialized equipment	Yes
Passive vs active treatment	Active requires engagement and adherence (practice and use of skills outside of sessions)	Active requires engagement and adherence (practice and use of skills outside of sessions)

HRV-BF has the least amount of sessions that yield clinical improvement, and it is relatively simple to integrate into a treatment session.[75] For example, it is feasible to include a brief session of HRV biofeedback and resonance frequency training with another evidence-based intervention to address symptoms of depression along with insomnia or as part of the relaxation-based treatment associated with CBT-I.[76] The option for group biofeedback may also improve accessibility.[77] As technology improves and becomes less expensive, these options may be more readily accessible in communities that might generally lack availability.

Telehealth

Biofeedback has traditionally occurred in the outpatient office setting in which either a technician or clinician is required to place electrodes or other instruments for monitoring physiologic functions in close proximity to the person receiving the treatment. Technological advances allow for home treatment, which may provide a critical opportunity in the current (pandemic) and future treatment landscape. Studies have described tele-neurofeedback options[29,78] and demonstrated feasibility.[29] Moreover, Krepel and colleagues demonstrated effectiveness of home-based SMR neurofeedback using a tele-neurofeedback device that improved sleep duration.[78] There are a multitude of devices and apps to engage in HRV biofeedback. Some

devices are small enough for daily travel and for discreet use in many settings. Biofeedback combined with CBT-I is a tool to address comorbidities and can easily occur as telehealth.

SUMMARY

Biofeedback uses various modalities to improve self-regulation and may reduce hyperarousal associated with insomnia. Biofeedback is a promising adjunct intervention to CBT-I despite concerns over research methodology. Biofeedback has demonstrated efficacy in a range of conditions frequently comorbid with insomnia. Given the high level of comorbidity of insomnia and other conditions, biofeedback may play an even more important role in addressing some of the limitations of CBT-I. Although CBT-I focuses on the perpetuating factors of insomnia, biofeedback can effectively address the precipitating factors. Additionally, for nonresponders to CBT-I, when it is contraindicated, or when it is not a desirable option, biofeedback may serve as an alternative intervention or used in combination with other common insomnia interventions.

FUTURE DIRECTIONS

Health-related sleep disparities are higher in communities of color.[79] Johnson and colleagues reviewed articles on racial and ethnic disparities and found that insomnia symptoms (ie, sleep duration, sleep quality, sleepiness, and sleep complaints) were generally worse in the representative sample of communities of color (eg, African Americans, Asians, Pacific Islanders) than in White samples. Billings and colleagues described interventions hypothesized to improve outcomes in sleep disparities and noted that discrimination in society increases stress and affect sleep. They hypothesized that culturally adapted interventions and empowerment might address sleep problems resulting from discrimination.[8] Jackson and colleagues described interventions to address sleep health disparities and suggested the importance of adapting and developing "evidence-based, culturally appropriate interventions across the life course for specific health disparity populations" (p.7).[80] Future studies may focus on the role of biofeedback interventions as a means of improving outcomes in sleep disparities via 2 pathways, increasing empowerment and reducing distress. First, empowerment is a concept that refers to among other things, increasing autonomy and power in traditionally marginalized communities.[81] Traditional psychological and medical interventions often use an approach that assumes the primary knowledge resides with the treating provider. By contrast, biofeedback may be viewed as an empowering intervention due to the collaborative relationship between provider and patient, as well as the active role of the patient in bringing about positive outcomes. This intervention allows the patient to learn about their physiology, implement self-regulatory strategies, and, through the use of feedback, see outcomes in real time. Second, biofeedback interventions improve self-regulation and parasympathetic responding with a goal of reducing overall distress.

There are several studies spanning decades that indicate positive outcomes using biofeedback for insomnia and other diagnoses. However, there is considerable debate about what constitutes rigorous research design in biofeedback and subsequent concern about placebo effects as the primary mechanism of biofeedback.[82] Nonspecific effects are readily capitalized on in biofeedback interventions and many of the reviews and some studies discount the value of these as part of the change process. For example, one recent neurofeedback study demonstrated the significant impact of participants' expectancy on perceptions of treatment efficacy in the absence of objective data.[83] Future research to consider the role and possible positive influence of unspecified elements, such as expectancy effects and motivation, elicited by biofeedback interventions in the treatment of insomnia is recommended.

Biofeedback interventions may facilitate engagement and adherence in the treatment of other disorders and the utilization of other modalities, including CBT-I. Other targets for biofeedback that are rarely measured in studies include increased self-efficacy that may benefit current and future treatment engagement and the transfer of treatment success to other relevant treatments. Other studies may wish to identify the disorders and populations for which biofeedback is more appropriate as an integrative intervention with CBT-I or preferred to CBT-I in the treatment of insomnia (**Table 1**).

CLINICS CARE POINTS

- Biofeedback offers a promising adjunct intervention or promising alternative when CBT-I is contraindicated or inadequate, as well as for those reluctant to engage in traditional psychotherapy or pharmacotherapy.
- Biofeedback has demonstrated effectiveness in the treatment of several disorders that frequently co-occur with insomnia.
- Biofeedback used as an adjunct to CBT-I may address some of the limitations of this standard treatment as well as hasten sleep gains.

DISCLOSURE

The authors have nothing to disclose.

REFERENCES

1. Blase K, Vermetten E, Lehrer P, et al. Neurophysiological approach by self-control of your stress-related autonomic nervous system with depression, stress and anxiety patients. Int J Environ Res Public Health 2021;18(7):3329.
2. Fournié C, Chouchou F, Dalleau G, et al. Heart rate variability biofeedback in chronic disease management: a systematic review. Complement Ther Med 2021;60:102750.
3. AAPB Website approved May 18 2008 (definition): Aapb.org. 2022. Home | AAPB. Available at: https://www.aapb.org/i4a/pages/index.cfm?pageid=1&pageid=3267. Accessed February 26, 2022.
4. Diagnostic and statistical manual of mental disorders: DSM-5™. 5th edition. Arlington: American Psychiatric Publishing, Inc.; 2013.
5. Ohayon MM. Epidemiology of insomnia: what we know and what we still need to learn. Sleep Med Rev 2002;6(2):97–111.

6. Buysse DJ, Angst J, Gamma A, et al. Prevalence, course, and comorbidity of insomnia and depression in young adults. Sleep 2008;31(4):473–80.

7. Morin CM, LeBlanc M, Daley M, et al. Epidemiology of insomnia: prevalence, self-help treatments, consultations, and determinants of help-seeking behaviors. Sleep Med 2006;7(2):123–30.

8. Billings ME, Cohen RT, Baldwin CM, et al. Disparities in sleep health and potential intervention models: a focused review. Chest 2021;159(3):1232–40.

9. Edinger JD, Arnedt JT, Bertisch SM, et al. Behavioral and psychological treatments for chronic insomnia disorder in adults: an American Academy of Sleep Medicine clinical practice guideline. J Clin Sleep Med 2021;17(2):255–62.

10. Cénat JM, Blais-Rochette C, Kokou-Kpolou CK, et al. Prevalence of symptoms of depression, anxiety, insomnia, posttraumatic stress disorder, and psychological distress among populations affected by the COVID-19 pandemic: a systematic review and meta-analysis. Psychiatry Res 2021;295:113599.

11. Wu T, Jia X, Shi H, et al. Prevalence of mental health problems during the COVID-19 pandemic: a systematic review and meta-analysis. J Affect Disord 2021;281:91–8.

12. Morin CM, Vézina-Im LA, Ivers H, et al. Prevalent, incident, and persistent insomnia in a population-based cohort tested before (2018) and during the first-wave of COVID-19 pandemic (2020). Sleep 2022;45(1):zsab258.

13. Jahrami H, BaHammam AS, Bragazzi NL, et al. Sleep problems during the COVID-19 pandemic by population: a systematic review and meta-analysis. J Clin Sleep Med 2021;17(2):299–313.

14. Irwin MR. Why sleep is important for health: a psychoneuroimmunology perspective. Annu Rev Psychol 2015;66:143–72.

15. Kessler RC, Berglund PA, Coulouvrat C, et al. Insomnia and the performance of US workers: results from the America insomnia survey. Sleep 2011;34(9):1161–71. published correction appears in Sleep. 2011;34(11):1608] [published correction appears in Sleep. 2012 Jun 1;35(6):725.

16. Trauer JM, Qian MY, Doyle JS, et al. Cognitive behavioral therapy for chronic insomnia: a systematic review and meta-analysis. Ann Intern Med 2015;163(3):191–204.

17. Qaseem A, Kansagara D, Forciea MA, et al. Clinical guidelines committee of the American College of Physicians. Management of chronic insomnia disorder in adults: a clinical practice guideline from the American College of Physicians. Ann Intern Med 2016;165(2):125–33.

18. Wu JQ, Appleman ER, Salazar RD, et al. Cognitive behavioral therapy for insomnia comorbid with psychiatric and medical conditions: a meta-analysis. JAMA Intern Med 2015;175(9):1461–72.

19. Smith MT, Huang MI, Manber R. Cognitive behavior therapy for chronic insomnia occurring within the context of medical and psychiatric disorders. Clin Psychol Rev 2005;25(5):559–92.

20. Tan G, Shaffer F, Lyle R, Teo I, editors. Evidence-Based Practice in Biofeedback and Neurofeedback. 3rd ed. Wheat Ridge, CO: Association of Applied Psychophysiology and Biofeedback; 2016.

21. Cho JH, Kremer S, Young J. Who to refer to a behavioral insomnia clinic? - recommendations based on treatment rationale and response prediction. Curr Sleep Med Rep 2021;1–8. https://doi.org/10.1007/s40675-021-00220-3. published online ahead of print, 2021 nov 17.

22. Buenaver LF, Townsend D, Ong JC. Delivering cognitive behavioral therapy for insomnia in the real world: considerations and controversies. Sleep Med Clin 2019;14(2):275–81.

23. Schwartz, M. Andrasik, F. Biofeedback. 3rd edition. New York: Guilford Press.

24. Monroe LJ. Psychological and physiological differences between good and poor sleepers. J Abnorm Psychol 1967;72(3):255–64.

25. Freedman R, Papsdorf JD. Biofeedback and progressive relaxation treatment of sleep-onset insomnia: a controlled, all-night investigation. Biofeedback Self Regul 1976;1(3):253–71.

26. Nicassio P, Bootzin R. A comparison of progressive relaxation and autogenic training as treatments for insomnia. J Abnorm Psychol 1974;83(3):253–60.

27. Dautovich ND, McNamara J, Williams JM, et al. Tackling sleeplessness: psychological treatment options for insomnia. Nat Sci Sleep 2010;2:23–37.

28. Hauri P. Treating psychophysiologic insomnia with biofeedback. Arch Gen Psychiatry 1981;38(7):752–8.

29. Hauri PJ, Percy L, Hellekson C, et al. The treatment of psychophysiologic insomnia with biofeedback: a replication study. Biofeedback Self Regul 1982;7(2):223–35.

30. Cortoos A, De Valck E, Arns M, et al. An exploratory study on the effects of tele-neurofeedback and tele-biofeedback on objective and subjective sleep in patients with primary insomnia. Appl Psychophysiol Biofeedback 2010;35(2):125–34.

31. Lovato N, Miller CB, Gordon CJ, et al. The efficacy of biofeedback for the treatment of insomnia: a critical review. Sleep Med 2019;56:192–200.

32. Arns M, Feddema I, Kenemans JL. Differential effects of theta/beta and SMR neurofeedback in ADHD on sleep onset latency. Front Hum Neurosci 2014;8:1019.

33. Gevirtz R. The promise of heart rate variability biofeedback: evidence-based applications. Appl Psychophysiol Biofeedback 2013;41(3):110–20.

34. Hasuo H, Kanbara K, Shizuma H, et al. Short-term efficacy of home-based heart rate variability

biofeedback on sleep disturbance in patients with incurable cancer: a randomised open-label study. BMJ Support Palliat Care 2020. https://doi.org/10.1136/bmjspcare-2020-002324.

35. Burch JB, Ginsberg JP, McLain AC, et al. Symptom management among cancer survivors: randomized pilot intervention trial of heart rate variability biofeedback. Appl Psychophysiol Biofeedback 2020;45(2):99–108.

36. Melo DLM, Carvalho LBC, Prado LBF, et al. Biofeedback therapies for chronic insomnia: a systematic review. Appl Psychophysiol Biofeedback 2019;44(4):259–69.

37. Lambert-Beaudet F, Journault WG, Rudziavic Provençal A, et al. Neurofeedback for insomnia: current state of research. World J Psychiatry 2021;11(10):897–914.

38. Kwan Y, Yoon S, Suh S, et al. A randomized controlled trial comparing neurofeedback and cognitive-behavioral therapy for insomnia patients: pilot study. Appl Psychophysiol Biofeedback 2022. https://doi.org/10.1007/s10484-022-09534-6. published online ahead of print, 2022 feb 11.

39. Lin IM, Fan SY, Yen CF, et al. Heart rate variability biofeedback increased autonomic Activation and improved symptoms of depression and insomnia among patients with major depression disorder. Clin Psychopharmacol Neurosci 2019;17(2):222–32. published correction appears in clin psychopharmacol neurosci. 2019 Aug 31;17(3):458.

40. Leem J, Cheong MJ, Lee H, et al. Effectiveness, cost-utility, and safety of neurofeedback self-regulating training in patients with post-traumatic stress disorder: a randomized controlled trial. Healthcare (Basel) 2021;9(10):1351.

41. Spielman AJ, Saskin P, Thorpy MJ. Treatment of chronic insomnia by restriction of time in bed. Sleep 1987;10(1):45–56.

42. Perlis ML, Pigeon WR, Grandner MA, et al. Why treat insomnia? J Prim Care Community Health 2021;12. https://doi.org/10.1177/21501327211014084. 21501327211014084.

43. Roth T. Comorbid insomnia: current directions and future challenges. Am J Manag Care 2009;15(Suppl):S6–13.

44. Pizzoli SFM, Marzorati C, Gatti D, et al. A meta-analysis on heart rate variability biofeedback and depressive symptoms. Sci Rep 2021;11(1):6650.

45. Arns M, Clark CR, Trullinger M, et al. Neurofeedback and Attention-deficit/hyperactivity-disorder (ADHD) in children: rating the evidence and proposed guidelines. Appl Psychophysiol Biofeedback 2020;45(2):39–48. https://doi.org/10.1007/s10484-020-09455-2.

46. Nagai M, Hoshide S, Kario K. Sleep duration as a risk factor for cardiovascular disease- a review of the recent literature. Curr Cardiol Rev 2010;6(1):54–61.

47. Burlacu A, Brinza C, Popa IV, et al. Influencing cardiovascular outcomes through heart rate variability modulation: a systematic review. Diagnostics (Basel) 2021;11(12):2198.

48. Ohayon MM, Roth T. Place of chronic insomnia in the course of depressive and anxiety disorders. J Psychiatr Res 2003;37(1):9–15.

49. Ramsawh HJ, Stein MB, Belik SL, et al. Relationship of anxiety disorders, sleep quality, and functional impairment in a community sample. J Psychiatr Res 2009;43(10):926–33.

50. Kushnir J, Marom S, Mazar M, et al. The link between social anxiety disorder, treatment outcome, and sleep difficulties among patients receiving cognitive behavioral group therapy. Sleep Med 2014;15(5):515–21.

51. Manber R, Carney C, Edinger J, et al. Dissemination of CBTI to the non-sleep specialist: protocol development and training issues. J Clin Sleep Med 2012;8(2):209–18.

52. Richards A, Kanady JC, Neylan TC. Sleep disturbance in PTSD and other anxiety-related disorders: an updated review of clinical features, physiological characteristics, and psychological and neurobiological mechanisms. Neuropsychopharmacology 2020;45(1):55–73. published correction appears in Neuropsychopharmacology. 2019 Oct 7.

53. Tolin DF, Davies CD, Moskow DM, et al. Biofeedback and neurofeedback for anxiety disorders: a quantitative and qualitative systematic review. Adv Exp Med Biol 2020;1191:265–89.

54. Lehrer P, Kaur K, Sharma A, et al. Heart rate variability biofeedback improves emotional and physical health and performance: a systematic review and meta analysis. Appl Psychophysiol Biofeedback 2020;45(3):109–29. published correction appears in Appl Psychophysiol Biofeedback. 2021 Dec;46(4):389.

55. Meuret AE, Rosenfield D, Seidel A, et al. Respiratory and cognitive mediators of treatment change in panic disorder: evidence for intervention specificity. J Consult Clin Psychol 2010;78(5):691–704.

56. Ross RJ, Ball WA, Sullivan KA, et al. Sleep disturbance as the hallmark of posttraumatic stress disorder. Am J Psychiatry 1989;146:697–707.

57. Maher MJ, Rego SA, Asnis GM. Sleep disturbances in patients with post-traumatic stress disorder: epidemiology, impact and approaches to management. CNS Drugs 2006;20(7):567–90.

58. Steingrimsson S, Bilonic G, Ekelund AC, et al. Electroencephalography-based neurofeedback as treatment for post-traumatic stress disorder: a systematic review and meta-analysis. Eur Psychiatry 2020;63(1):e7.

59. Soehner AM, Kaplan KA, Harvey AG. Prevalence and clinical correlates of co-occurring insomnia

and hypersomnia symptoms in depression. J Affect Disord 2014;167:93–7.

60. Khurshid KA. Comorbid insomnia and psychiatric disorders: an update. Innov Clin Neurosci 2018; 15(3–4):28–32.

61. Stewart R, Besset A, Bebbington P, et al. Insomnia comorbidity and impact and hypnotic use by age group in a national survey population aged 16 to 74 years. Sleep 2006;29(11):1391–7.

62. Davydov DM, Shapiro D, Cook IA, et al. Baroreflex mechanisms in major depression. Prog Neuropsychopharmacol Biol Psychiatry 2007;31(1):164–77.

63. Sgoifo A, Carnevali L, Alfonso Mde L, et al. Autonomic dysfunction and heart rate variability in depression. Stress 2015;18(3):343–52.

64. Walker BF. The prevalence of low back pain: a systematic review of the literature from 1966 to 1998. J Spinal Disord 2000;13(3):205–17.

65. Haack M, Simpson N, Sethna N, et al. Sleep deficiency and chronic pain: potential underlying mechanisms and clinical implications. Neuropsychopharmacology 2020;45(1):205–16.

66. Tang NK. Insomnia co-occurring with chronic pain: clinical features, interaction, assessments and possible interventions. Rev Pain 2008;2(1):2–7.

67. Lehrer PM, Gevirtz R. Heart rate variability biofeedback: how and why does it work? Front Psychol 2014;5:756.

68. Reneau M. Heart rate variability biofeedback to treat fibromyalgia: an integrative literature review. Pain Manag Nurs 2020;21(3):225–32.

69. Quigg M, Gharai S, Ruland J, et al. Insomnia in epilepsy is associated with continuing seizures and worse quality of life. Epilepsy Res 2016;122:91–6.

70. Sterman MB. Basic concepts and clinical findings in the treatment of seizure disorders with EEG operant conditioning. Clin Electroencephalogr 2000;31(1): 45–55.

71. Viola-Saltzman M, Musleh C. Traumatic brain injury-induced sleep disorders. Neuropsychiatr Dis Treat 2016;12:339–48.

72. Ludwig R, Vaduvathiriyan P, Siengsukon C. Does cognitive-behavioural therapy improve sleep outcomes in individuals with traumatic brain injury: a scoping review. Brain Inj 2020;34(12):1569–78.

73. Baker VB, Eliasen KM, Hack NK. Lifestyle modifications as therapy for medication refractory post-traumatic headache (PTHA) in the military population of Okinawa. J Headache Pain 2018;19(1):113.

74. Rosenthal R. New guidelines for third party reimbursement for biofeedback. association for applied psychophysiology and biofeedback. Available at: https://www.aapb.org/i4a/pages/index.cfm? pageid=3387. Accessed February 26, 2022.

75. Schoenberg PL, David AS. Biofeedback for psychiatric disorders: a systematic review. Appl Psychophysiol Biofeedback 2014;39(2):109–35.

76. Caldwell YT, Steffen PR. Adding HRV biofeedback to psychotherapy increases heart rate variability and improves the treatment of major depressive disorder. Int J Psychophysiol 2018;131:96–101.

77. Fischer CJ, Moravec CS, Khorshid L. The "How and Why" of Group biofeedback for chronic disease management. Appl Psychophysiol Biofeedback 2018;43(4):333–40.

78. Krepel N, Egtberts T, Touré-Cuq E, et al. Evaluation of the URGOnight tele-neurofeedback device: an open-label feasibility study with follow-up. Appl Psychophysiol Biofeedback 2021. https://doi.org/10. 1007/s10484-021-09525-z. published online ahead of print, 2021 sep 28.

79. Johnson DA, Jackson CL, Williams NJ, et al. Are sleep patterns influenced by race/ethnicity - a marker of relative advantage or disadvantage? Evidence to date. Nat Sci Sleep 2019;11:79–95.

80. Jackson CL, Walker JR, Brown MK, et al. A workshop report on the causes and consequences of sleep health disparities. Sleep 2020; 43(8):zsaa037.

81. Halvorsen K, Dihle A, Hansen C, et al. Empowerment in healthcare: a thematic synthesis and critical discussion of concept analyses of empowerment. Patient Educ Couns 2020;103(7):1263–71.

82. Pigott HE, Cannon R, Trullinger M. The fallacy of sham-controlled neurofeedback trials: a reply to thibault and colleagues (2018). J Atten Disord 2021; 25(3):448–57.

83. Schönenberg M, Weingärtner AL, Weimer K, et al. Believing is achieving - on the role of treatment expectation in neurofeedback applications. Prog Neuropsychopharmacol Biol Psychiatry 2021;105: 110129.

Hypnotic Medications as an Adjunct Treatment to Cognitive Behavioral Therapy for Insomnia

Paul Barkopoulos, MD, MPH[a,b,*], Joshua Hyong-Jin Cho, MD, PhD[a]

KEYWORDS

- Adjunctive • Augmentation • Cognitive behavioral treatment for insomnia • Combination • Hypnotic
- Insomnia • Pharmacotherapy • Adjunct

KEY POINTS

- Theoretic rationale and randomized controlled trial (RCT) results support consideration of combining hypnotics and cognitive behavioral therapy for insomnia (CBT-I), (combination of hypnotics and CBT-I abbreviated as COMB hereafter), as an appropriate adaptation to CBT-I for insomnia patients needing a more rapid onset in perceived sleep improvement while still allowing them to attain the posttreatment durability of benefit that CBT-I can afford.
- Full-component CBT-I monotherapy should continue to be promoted as the initial treatment of choice for almost all patients, as even patients with pretreatment risk factors for suboptimal CBT-I response may still remit with monotherapy.
- COMB RCTs suggest that an intermediate half-life hypnotic such as zolpidem will not confer appreciable harm to patients' short- and long-term outcomes, as compared with CBT-I monotherapy. COMB does not seem to confer an increased risk for hypnotic dependence, misuse, or abuse short or long term.
- No pretreatment patient characteristics, such as short sleep duration, low sleep efficiency, psychiatric comorbidity, daytime symptoms, or insomnia phenotype, should be relied on in order to make treatment decisions regarding COMB. However, such risk factors for CBT-I suboptimal response can serve to increase clinician alertness for signs of impending attrition or non-remission during the course of CBT-I.
- COMB is best instituted early during the course of CBT-I, within the first 4 weeks, whereupon the risk for attrition is highest.
- RCT findings suggest that adjunctive hypnotics should and can be tapered quickly before the termination of CBT-I in order to optimize outcomes.
- As higher sleep quality (SQ) scores assessed using sleep diary just prior to, or after, a CBT-I session are associated with increased adherence, low scores that fail to improve, especially early during those first few weeks of CBT-I, may serve as a potentially sensitive marker for beneficial COMB intervention.

[a] Department of Psychiatry and Biobehavioral Sciences, David Geffen School of Medicine at UCLA, UCLA Insomnia Clinic, Cousins Center for Psychoneuroimmunology, University of California Los Angeles, 300 Medical Plaza Driveway, Los Angeles, CA, 90025, USA; [b] Cedars Sinai Medical Center, 8700 Beverly Blvd #2900A, Los Angeles, CA, 90048, USA
* Corresponding author. 1800 Fairburn Avenue, Suite 108, Los Angeles, CA 90025.
E-mail address: pbarkopoulos@mednet.ucla.edu

Sleep Med Clin 18 (2023) 95–111
https://doi.org/10.1016/j.jsmc.2022.10.004
1556-407X/23/© 2022 Elsevier Inc. All rights reserved.

INTRODUCTION

Chronic insomnia disorder, for our purposes, insomnia disorder (ID), is defined broadly as difficulty in initiating or maintaining sleep that occurs at least 3 nights out of the week for 3 months. ID is a highly recalcitrant and impactful disease.[1,2] Left untreated, ID is associated with significant impairments in daytime function,[3] safety (vehicle and occupational accidents),[4–6] and increased risks for developing medical and psychiatric illnesses.[7–9] Despite the enormous direct and indirect costs exacted by ID worldwide, only two treatments for ID, cognitive behavioral therapy for insomnia (CBT-I) and hypnotic pharmacotherapy (PCT), are supported by the American Academy of Sleep Medicine (AASM)[10,11] as being sufficient evidenced-based to allow for their recommendation. Of the two, CBT-I has become the treatment of first choice due to its established capacity to effect both safe and sustainable longer term outcomes.[12] However, ID is a complex and heterogeneous disease, and CBT-I, laudable a treatment as it is, will not help all patients, leaving the potentially indefinite provision of PCT as the only option left for patients.[1] This narrative review will attempt to provide a clinical rationale for the adjunctive use of hypnotics along with CBT-I (the combination of PCT and CBT-I abbreviated as COMB hereafter) as an alternative treatment option based on theoretical evidence in conjunction with findings derived from select RCTs that compare COMB directly with CBT-I. From such a synthesis, treatment suggestions will be offered that can hopefully help guide clinicians in COMB-related decision-making.

NATURE OF THE PROBLEM
Adequacy of Evidence-Based Insomnia Disorder Treatments: CBT-I versus Pharmacotherapy on the Optimal Treatment Scorecard

Acute remission
Being mindful that remission, not response, is the holy grail of outcomes for chronic illness, monotherapy study comparisons suggest that both CBT-I and PCT produce comparable rates of remission, approximating 40% (remission based on validated insomnia symptom scales (such as the widely accepted Insomnia Severity Index [ISI][13]).[2,14,15]

Treatment burden
PCT is clearly more accessible and requires less patient effort and is less costly short term, than CBT-I. However, PCT can cause severe adverse events such as complex sleep-related behaviors (CSRBs)[16] and increase the risk for accidents[17] and falls.[10,18–20] CBT-I can also instigate troublesome side effects early in treatment, due mostly to the acute impact of the sleep restriction (SRT) component contained within CBT-I. [21–23]These side effects can include increases in daytime somnolence, fatigue, irritability, cognitive, and psychomotor dysfunction.[21,22] However, significant safety-related adverse events due to CBT-I appear rare.

Attrition/adherence
Although attrition rates for CBT-I seem to be low in randomized controlled trials (RCTs), approximating 8% for both treatment and active controls.[24] general sleep clinic population dropout rates can range from 9.7% to 38.8%.[25] Data is lacking regarding attrition to PCT treatment in the general ID population.

Recurrence prevention and durability of benefit
ID is a highly recurrent disease if left untreated.[26] CBT-I does evidence the capacity to provide sustained benefit years after treatment termination.[27,28] No such evidence exists for PCT. ID seems to recur at a high rate upon PCT discontinuation.[26,27] As well, PCT benefits seem to degrade over time.[27] It is here that CBT-I may most distinguish itself on the optimal treatment scorecard. Few acute treatments for chronic illnesses can claim both relief of symptoms and inoculation against recurrence of future episodes.

Sleep parameter improvement
Objectively measured sleep outcomes using polysomnography (PSG) or actigraphy demonstrate that CBT-I and PCT are effective in acutely lowering sleep onset latency (SOL) and wakefulness after sleep onset (WASO), but CBT-I tends to incite a negative impact on total sleep time (TST). TST often declines below baseline for much of the course of CBT-I.[21] PCT is more effective at acutely increasing TST.[7–9,18,21,28–30]

Improvements in daytime insomnia disorder symptoms
Remarkably, little information is available from PCT studies that address daytime improvements. CBT-I can improve all daytime symptoms associated with ID, but that journey may be slow, with some studies reporting that it can take weeks to achieve improvement in fatigue, somnolence, and cognitive function from baseline levels.[31,32] Both treatments, when they confer remission in ID, can beneficially impact depression and anxiety symptoms.[33–37]

Trajectory of benefit
PCT RCT data support that the onset of subjectively and objectively measured sleep improvements can occur rapidly. For CBT-I, perceived benefits may take weeks.[28]

Secondary favorable long-term outcomes
Any potential longer term benefit with PCT requires sustained application. As such, safety risks associated with PCT do not abate and can increase as tolerance develops along with potential dose escalation. As well, the risk for pharmaceutical-related adverse events increases as people age. CBT-I, unlike PCT, allows patients to resolve perpetuating factors that maintain ID and, as such, does not require continuous provision of treatment, undoubtedly the safest strategy long term. As well, because ID tends to be a bidirectional illness[38] that is impacted by and directly impacts other illnesses. Improvement in ID from either CBT-I or PCT[33,39,40] may benefit other health outcomes, such as major depressive disorder (MDD) remission and recurrence.[15,38,41]

Efficacy across subpopulations
A recently published 2020 AASM practice guideline, utilizing the rigorous Grading of Recommendations Assessment, Development and Evaluation (GRADE) process methodology for vetting the available literature,[12] has provided evidence-based support for CBT-I as an efficacious treatment not only for primary ID, but also for ID comorbid with medical and psychiatric illness.[38,42] Full multicomponent CBT-I was the only behavioral treatment (BT) afforded a maximum STRONG recommendation from the AASM. CBT-I also demonstrates efficacy in treating older patients[1,43,44] and may assist hypnotic-dependent patients in tapering off medication, and in reducing or eliminating future use.[45–47] Such data is lacking for PCT.

Optimal treatment scorecard conclusions
The bad news for treating ID is that both CBT-I and PCT will leave a substantial proportion of patients who undertake either treatment with continuing symptoms (non-remission). On the positive side, CBT-I provides several evidence-based optimal treatment qualities, especially that of offering a maintained remission long after active treatment concludes, without reliance on medications. However, patients must first achieve remission before they can sustain it. CBT-I could use some help with remission rates so that more patients can appreciate such longer term benefits.

THEORETIC RATIONALE SUPPORTING COMB
Improving Insomnia Disorder Outcomes by Adding Adjunctive Treatments to Cognitive Behavioral Therapy for Insomnia

The remaining sections of this article will be based on the conceptual premise that full multicomponent CBT-I, a treatment paradigm years in the making that evidences several optimal treatment features, including its capacity to confer a durable posttreatment remission, should serve as the basic template for building even more effective ID treatments. Such a concept has been widely endorsed, as much investigation is being devoted to testing various adaptations to CBT-I that also involve addition of other treatments,[48] such as transcranial magnetic stimulation,[49] hypnosis,[50] bright light,[18,51] and mindfulness.[25] Of note, all such treatments possess less evidence supporting their efficacy as a primary treatment for ID than does PCT.

Acceptable Efficacy Versus Harm Profile of Pharmacotherapy for COMB Purposes

Balancing efficacy and safety
Treatments that possess an established evidence basis for balancing efficacy and safety as a monotherapy for ID should serve as particularly promising candidates for CBT-I add-on. As a key objective of COMB would be to get more ID patients to remit with CBT-I so that they can actualize a future with less reliance on PCT, COMB for the purposes of this article is envisioned as a targeted and time-limited augmentation strategy. PCT would be ideally discontinued before the termination of CBT-I. Subsequently, the following discussion regarding risk–benefit considerations will focus on evidence derived mostly from short duration PCT studies (4–12 weeks).

The 2017 AASM pharmacologic practice guidelines (GRADE)[10] has afforded only certain hypnotics a proactive recommendation, that is, better to use than not. These hypnotics include three benzodiazepine receptor agonists (BZRAs or Z drugs), zaleplon, zolpidem, zolpidem er, and eszopiclone; two benzodiazepines (BZDs) triazolam and temazepam, one antihistamine, doxepin; one melatonin receptor antagonist, ramelteon; and one dual orexin receptor antagonist (DORA), suvorexant (noting that the recently released lemborexant was not available when the AASM 2017 investigation was conducted). However, only zolpidem, zolpidem er, eszopiclone, and temazepam are recommended for ID patients presenting with both difficulty in initiating and maintaining sleep. As most ID patients suffer from both problems,[28] PCT that provides an evidence-based broad spectrum of efficacy is most appropriate for COMB purposes. Discussion will be restricted further to the two BZRAs: zolpidem and eszopiclone. Although controversial, BZRAs possess properties that may offer advantages over older BZDs.[52] Also, BZRAs are the pharmaceuticals most examined in contemporary ID research, including the COMB RCTs pending our discussion..

Benzodiazepine receptor agonist short-term safety

BZRAs were developed as an alternative to BZDs as they provide targeted agonism of GABA-A receptor delta 1-subunits, as opposed to BZDs, which are full GABA-agonists. A less debatable advantage for BZRAs is that they possess much shorter half-lives than BZDs (1 hour for zaleplon, 1.5–4.5 hours for zolpidem and zolpidem er, and 6 hours for eszopiclone[5,7,11], as contrasted to temazepam with a half life around 15 hours). Being mindful that approximately five (5) half-lives are required to totally eliminate a person's blood of all traces of medication, a short half-life hypnotic is less likely intrude its sedative action into active daytime hours.[2,5,7,11] As well, BZRAs demonstrate minimal alteration of sleep stage architecture. Both BZRAs and BZDs confer a rapid dose-proportional therapeutic effect, allowing for pinpoint dose titration for individual patients.[7] BZRAs seem to have little potential for respiratory suppression and toxicity at recommended doses.[53,54]

Despite these positive qualities, and although a meta-analysis of U.S. Food and Drug Administration (FDA) approval RCTs did not demonstrate serious adverse events due to BZRAs,[55] these agents can induce significant negative side effects, the most ominous being CSRBs, which earned them a black box warning from the FDA in 2019. As well, BZRAs can incite parasomnias, amnesia, and increase the risk for falls and injury, particularly when ambulation occurs in the middle of the night. As noted, such risks, including that for CSRBs, persist as hypnotic use continues, and will increase as people age.[2,10,56]

Dependence, abuse, and misuse

CBT-I holds out the promise of providing a remission that does not rely on pharmaceuticals. Understandably, using a hypnotic to enhance response to CBT-I elicits concern about doing just the opposite, inducing dependence on the augmenting agent. One recent prospective investigation reported that one out of five first-time users of PCT will become long-term (1 year) users, though only 0.5% of PCT users will engage in excessive use[118]. It is here that it may be important to distinguish between dependence, misuse, and abuse. Misuse is defined as using a medication in a manner that was not intended for the illness, such as taking extra zolpidem for an awakening in the middle of the night. Abuse involves the use of medication for nonmedical reasons, such as obtaining recreational effects. Physiologic dependence requires that the medication induce tolerance and withdrawal upon abrupt discontinuation (Rebound, unrelated to whether a medication causes tolerance or not, describes the spring back of disease-related symptoms to greater than baseline levels when a dose is missed or blood levels decline.) BZDs, BZRAs, and DORAs are listed as U.S. Drug Enforcement Agency (DEA) schedule 4 agents, which indicates that they confer modest reinforcing effects and thus are potentially liable for abuse. Abuse and overdose toxicity for BZRAs generally occurs in conjunction with more powerful euphorigenic substances, particularly alcohol or stimulants, a problem largely incurred by substance use disorder (SUD) patients.[57,58] Like BZDs, BZRAs possess the chemical capacity to produce tolerance, which can propel dose escalation, which then increases the risk for a dose-dependent withdrawal. This risk seems lower for BZRAs than BZDs, potentially related to lower BZRA propensity to deform the GABA receptor.[59] Clinically, short-term controlled studies reviewed by the AASM do not evidence significant tolerance, rebound, or withdrawal due to BZRAs,[10] and a 12 month RCT involving zolpidem indicated no rebound signals.[60]

COMB risk–benefit determination

Ultimately, the use of PCT must be weighed against the risk of the disease. As pertinent to COMB, the dangers of a strategically targeted limited application of a BZRA in conjunction with CBT-I must be considered relative to the dangers of unremitted ID. Residual ID symptoms increase the risk for recurrence of fully syndromic ID.[61] Persisting ID symptoms are themselves associated with several negative consequences, including increased motor vehicle accidents,[5,62–64] cognitive dysfunction,[65] mood impairment,[66] falls and hip fracture,[67] and suicidality.[68] Short sleep duration ID may be especially pernicious and has been connected to numerous short- and long-term adverse health consequences,[69] including an increased association with daytime cognitive and motor dysfunction.[21,23,29,70] As well, persistent ID is indirectly associated with the increased use of psychoactive substances,[65,71] including alcohol, the most widely used hypnotic. The importance of carefully assessing relative risk is exemplified by an elegant RCT[72] that compared 12 months of blinded patient-controlled dosing of either zolpidem or placebo. Over time, subjects receiving placebo tended toward greater escalation of their doses than did zolpidem recipients. In short, inadequately treated ID conferred a greater risk for misuse of PCT than did tolerance to zolpidem. In conclusion, non-remission of ID subsequent to CBT-I should be avoided, and the clinician should be prepared to offer more assertive options for their patients who appear headed in that direction.

Risk mitigation

Monotherapy studies support that many adverse events connected to BZRAs, including misuse and abuse of these agents, can be mitigated by a best practice approach.[10] Effective adverse event reduction starts with a comprehensive sleep and medical evaluation that thoroughly accounts for modifiable and non-modifiable risk factors that can increase the propensity for treatment-related adverse events, including older age, history of adverse events, substance and alcohol use, cognitive dysfunction, number of coexisting prescription and over-the-counter medications, medical and psychiatric comorbidity, potential for drug–drug interactions, and low psychosocial support.[11] As noted, the occurrence of BZRA-related adverse events is proportional to the number of coexisting medications and substances. As such, treatment-related adverse events can be preempted by attentiveness to such modifiable risk factors. High-risk patients, such as those with a prior history of active substance or alcohol use disorder, should likely not receive BZRAs. Patient education and informed consent are critical, as early signs of emerging adverse events can be detected by the patient or caregiver and reported to the clinician, which can then prompt the undertaking of actionable mitigation measures. Such proactive steps can include dose adjustments (start low, go slow), pill counts, limiting the numbers of pills prescribed, and the deprescribing[73] of unnecessary medications.

Increased frequency of follow-up visits is clearly associated with a reduction in treatment-related adverse events.[10,11] The AASM 2017 practice guidelines state "Even longer term BZRA prescribing may be largely safe under properly controlled circumstances." The argument could be made that an index course of CBT-I actually provides a most ideal outpatient vehicle for the optimal supervision of PCT due to a built in structure of weekly face-to-face personalized ID-focused sessions.

Consideration of Pharmacotherapy Interference with the Beneficial Mechanism of Cognitive Behavioral Therapy for Insomnia

Surprisingly, the mechanisms by which CBT-I confers long-term benefit remain unclear. One reasonable overall assumption is that successful CBT-I requires new learning. Some literature has implicated BZDs as interfering with the acquisition of fear extinction learning believed to be essential for the success of exposure-based interventions for conditions such as PTSD and social anxiety. It has been suggested that GABA-active agents similar to BZDs, such as BZRAs, may do the same. However, the evidence supporting BZD interference with exposure-based interventions is conflicted, as some meta-analyses support an interference,[74] whereas others conclude no interference, or even a benefit to combining BZDs.[75] As well, the question as to how BZRAs might infect learning that occurs during times when the drug is inactive, such as when CBT-I sessions are delivered, remains unanswered.

It has also been suggested that PCT might interfere with theorized psychological mediators necessary for positive CBT-I outcomes, such as attaining an improved sense of self-efficacy.[76] Self-efficacy is defined as confidence in one's ability to navigate a problem. Some studies demonstrate that ID improvement with PCT does not improve self-efficacy.[14] However, going back to the point of avoiding non-remission, it could be postulated that failing a course of CBT-I would do little to enhance self-efficacy actualization.

How Pharmacotherapy May Enhance Cognitive Behavioral Therapy for Insomnia: Possible Mechanisms of Action

Understanding what patient- and treatment-related factors confer problems for CBT-I can allow for theoretic assumptions as to how PCT, in this case a BZRA, based on its clinical profile and mechanism of action, could further buttress CBT-I.

Pretreatment patient characteristics associated with suboptimal CBT-I treatment response, as well as poor adherence, include psychopathology (higher depression and anxiety), hypnotic dependence, short duration sleep,[77] and daytime fatigue.[21,22,78] Improving the tolerability or trajectory of benefit for CBT-I might tip the scale for some patients who might might discontinue or disengage from treatment. Several targets have been proposed whereby BZRAs could compensate for CBT-Is lack of fit for such patients.

Sleep restriction and total sleep time

SRT is associated with the acute onset of daytime adverse effects such as fatigue and sleepiness. Concurrent with the onset of these side effects, SRT is precipitating a decline in TST. Although TST slowly recovers from its initial slide later in the course of CBT-I, and can actually further improve after CBT-I discontinuation as patients continue to increase their time in bed (TIB), some vulnerable patients will never get to that point. Short sleep diary-reported TST (<3.65 hours) has been associated with a 60% dropout rate in a general sleep clinic population before the 4th week of CBT-I.[25]

Fatigue, the most commonly occurring SRT-induced daytime symptom,[22] has been associated with increased attrition.[21,78,79] Modafinil, a stimulant, was demonstrated in one small trial to relieve SRT-related fatigue, relief that was associated with improved adherence to CBT-I.[79,119] Unfortunately, no data exists regarding improvement in SRT related ID fatigue with PCT.

Unlike CBT-I, PCT can rapidly improve objectively all sleep parameters,[7] including lengthening TST. Also, based on the analyses of comparative monotherapy study results, PCT tends to confer an earlier onset of subjective improvement in sleep than do BTs.[80]

In conclusion, PCTs rapid positive effect on TST could blunt the acute degradation of TST caused by SRT, potentially improving adherence to CBT-I.

Objective short duration sleep and insomnia disorder phenotype
Short sleep duration in general has been associated with suboptimal CBT-I treatment response.[77] ID with objectively measured short sleep duration has been advocated as an even more specific clinical marker than sleep diary-reported TST in predicting CBT-I treatment intolerance and suboptimal response.

Vgontzas[81] has lead the charge in proposing an ID phenotype hypothesis that is headlined by objective short sleep duration. Insomnia with short sleep duration (ISSD) is characterized by an average baseline TST <6 hour using PSG (or less precisely using actigraphy).[29,82] Insomnia with normal sleep duration is characterized by an average baseline TST ≥6 hr. Three RCTs have supported a blunted response to CBT-I for ISSD,[82] but four other studies did not support a diminished response to CBT-I.[83] However, it should be noted that these studies vary widely in methodology. Most germane to this discussion is the notion that a compromised TST would be a most amenable target for COMB.

Psychopathology such as depression and anxiety
As noted, psychopathologic daytime clinical features have been associated with suboptimal response to CBT-I and could serve as potential markers for COMB targeting. Both depression and anxiety are bidirectionally connected with

ID.[36,84–87] Thus, improvement (or worsening) in one illness can help (or hinder) the other, although, importantly, as an independent illness, remission to ID does not confer remission to a connected illness.[88] Results from the recently published REST-IT trial support how the treatment of ID with a BZRA can improve daytime depressive symptomology.[85] Zolpidem, when provided for SSRI-treated MDD/ID comorbid patients, was significantly more effective than placebo in reducing suicidality. Prior studies support that ID improvements conferred by both CBT-I and PCT monotherapies can assist with daytime depressive and anxiety symptoms.[33,41,86] In conclusion, addition of a BZRA to CBT-I could be a most effective strategy for addressing CBT-I treatment resistance that occurs for patients exhibiting higher psychopathology.

Hyperarousal
All ID seems to be associated with abnormal hyperarousal. ID patients display trait markers of daytime hyperarousal, such as increased scores on the multiple sleep latency test (MSLT) versus non-ID sufferers. This seems to explain why ID patients infrequently present with daytime somnolence. Theorists propose that dysfunctional hyperarousal underpins why ID sufferers have difficulty in obtaining the healthy sleep that "good sleepers" enjoy. Although what exactly constitutes good sleep biologically is not well established, normal sleepers, based on electroencephalographic (EEG) findings, experience approximately 90-min recurring sleep cycles that balance rapid eye movement (REM) with deeper non-rapid eye movement (NREM) stages[110]. When these cycles run uninterrupted throughout the night, people achieve adequate immersion in each sleep stage, all of which are essential. Excessive arousal, emanating from wakefulness centers in the brain, is postulated to intrude inappropriately on the NREM sleep of ID patients, as reflected by the increased presence of fast wave activity (increased sleep spindles, K complexes, and Beta power). Theoretically, such a mixing of sleep and wake disrupts a normal progression through sleep stages, forcing repeated reboots.[38,111,89] ID patients may be less able to effectively pass through lighter NREM stages 1 and 2 in order to attain sufficient time in deeper NREM sleep stages 3 and 4.[89] It is also theorized that such deficits occur within the microstructure of sleep, whereby greater neurobiological vulnerability for certain ID patients resides. SRT, a potent treatment, can potentially induce hyper-activation in susceptible people, a concept represented by disorders that are considered contraindications for SRT such as

bipolar I and epilepsy[90] and perhaps attention deficit hyperactivity disorder (ADHD)[91]

Increased hyperarousal vulnerability theory might explain how certain conditions which confer increased resistance to, or intolerance of CBT-I, mechanistically tie together. This list includes the aforementioned psychopathology (One study demonstrating that higher anxiety and MSLT scores were proportionally associated with increasing prescription hypnotic use)[115], short sleep, obstructive sleep apnea (OSA), periodic limb movement disorder, restless leg syndrome, and akathisia.[116] Fragmented sleep and low sleep efficiency (SE), has been associated, independently from TST, with adverse daytime outcomes such as falls in older adults[92–94] and blunted responses to CBT-I.[82] As noted, the objective short sleep phenotype ISSD is thought to represent a more hyper-aroused ID patient that exhibits elevations in peripheral markers of hypothalamic pituitary axis activation, such as cortisol.[9,81] Phenotype theorists are incorporating other novel clinical indicators of aberrant hyperarousal, such as within sleep reactivity,[114] that might help to direct treatment. Although CBT-I may eventually lessen brain hyperarousal[117], it does not do so acutely. However, GABA agonists, such as BZRAs, do so immediately, as well as lowering some markers of more broadly based hyperarousal.

Brain GABAergic dysfunction[95] may be central to unleashing unrestricted arousal contamination of sleep. BZRAs inhibit arousal emanating from brain wakefulness centers.[84,96] They are conjectured to improve sleep continuity on EEG and strengthen the "flip flop switch" that moves REM and NREM sleep smoothly back and forth.[89] BZRAs increase beneficial delta power and mitigate fast wave activity on EEG.[89] BZRAs can decrease hypoxemia and apneas in subsets of OSA and central sleep apnea patients that share impaired brain arousal regulation over sleep and breathing similar to that which occurs for ID patients without disordered breathing,[112,76,97,98] that benefit even extending to some opioid-dependent patients[113]. Studies indicate that BZRAs can increase continuous positive airway pressure (CPAP) adherence[99] and decrease snoring in middle-aged women.[100] BZRAs at standard doses are conjectured to increase the arousal threshold just enough to prevent microarousals that lead to breathing disruption, but not enough to decrease respiratory drive.

In conclusion, certain clinical pretreatment and within-treatment indicators of excessive hyperarousal could serve as potential targets for the compensatory arousal reduction that COMB could provide.

Psychological targets

Psychological factors seem to be mediators of successful outcomes with CBT-I, such as the previously mentioned sense of self-efficacy. It has been proposed that patients who succeed with CBT-I are able to cross an important threshold later in treatment whereby they start to identify themselves as "good sleepers."[21] A meta-analysis by Mellor[101] of CBT-I adherence studies concluded that one of the most consistent predictors of positive adherence to CBT-I was the patient's subjective experience of better sleep, based on sleep diary-reported sleep quality (SQ), on nights pre- and post-CBT-I session. It has been proposed that CBT-I treatment-resistant patients may be neurobiologically less able to perceive an improvement in sleep.[102] Such patients may be in particular need of a "good night's sleep" that can be connected to their CBT-I treatment, which could provide reinforcement for completing fully their remaining sessions.

COMB RANDOMIZED CONTROLLED TRIAL EVIDENCE: REVIEW OF SEMINAL STUDIES

There are surprisingly few RCTs that directly compare COMB with CBT-I or integrate CBT-I and PCT monotherapy in some fashion. However, even one well-designed RCT can provide a higher level of evidence that could help confirm or contradict theoretical assumptions derived from volumes of monotherapy and bench science research. RCT findings could be helpful not only in supporting whether COMB offers any advantage over CBT-I in regard to short- or long-term outcomes, but also provide some insights into clinical decision-making particulars.

Morin and colleagues, 1999: Morin and colleagues[20] have been responsible for most of the substantive short- and long-term COMB controlled outcome data generated in the twenty-first century. Though pre-2000, this seminal 1999 study is still worth mentioning because its findings remain relevant to the current practice of CBT-I. Of note, comparisons included not only COMB and CBT-I arms, but also PCT and placebo controls, a rarity in more modern RCTs. Results at 6 weeks and 2 years post demonstrated that subjects receiving COMB consisting of CBT-I and temazepam (a BZD) experienced the greatest number of benefits over time while those receiving temazepam alone regressed to pretreatment levels of ID symptomology. Improvements were more rapid for subjects receiving COMB or temazepam versus CBT-I monotherapy. The central conclusion culminating from Morin 1999 was that certain ID patients could experience both the rapid relief of symptoms provided by PCT as well as the longer term gains afforded by CBT-I when both treatments were combined acutely.

Jacobs and colleagues 2004[103]: This small 6-week RCT used a similar four-arm design as did Morin 1999, comparing zolpidem-based COMB, PCT, CBT-I, and placebo treatments for subjects specifically suffering from sleep initiation insomnia. Results revealed that both COMB and CBT-I were significantly more effective than PCT or placebo. CBT-I alone seemed most effective at getting patients to achieve near normative sleep thresholds of greater than 80% SE and less than 30 min SOL at 3 months post.

Vallieres and colleagues, 2005[104]: This small sequential crossover study compared treatments using zopiclone, a BZRA. Sequences starting with COMB when switched over to CBT-I demonstrated a protective effect for COMB against the subsequent degradation of TST induced by CBT-I monotherapy. COMB also provided a more rapid trajectory of response than did CBT-I. At 3 months, CBT-I monotherapy seemed to catch up to COMB, such that COMB did not evidence an advantage over the longer term.

Morin and colleagues, 2009[1]: This study remains the most substantive RCT involving COMB to date; 242 patients were randomized to a 6-week first-stage treatment of either CBT-I or COMB using zolpidem. After 6 weeks, CBT-I monotherapy patients were then randomized to either stage two 6-month extended CBT-I treatment or no treatment, whereas COMB patients were randomized to either CBT-I extension with as-needed zolpidem (maximum ten 10 mg pills per month) or CBT-I extension with no as-needed hypnotic. Results revealed that stage 1 COMB subjects were significantly more able to achieve ISI-determined remission after stage two 6-month treatment and at 1 year post-index treatment. COMB patients allowed no hypnotic in extended treatment maintained remission better than COMB subjects allowed as-needed zolpidem during extended treatment. Although COMB and CBT-I performed equally well regarding response and remission after stage 1 treatment, COMB was associated with significantly larger improvements in TST than was CBT-I (difference 15.9 min). No differences in attrition were noted between groups. Pill counts confirmed that subjects receiving as-needed zolpidem in extension only used on average one-half of their 10-pill allotment.

A post hoc analysis of this 2009 study data[105] addressed 1-year and 2-year outcomes for all treatment arms. COMB trended toward the greatest level of sustained remission, compared with CBT-I monotherapy groups, though COMB subjects who received as-needed zolpidem during 6-month extension maintained their benefits the least. Interestingly, COMB patients without as-needed zolpidem also tended toward less prescription hypnotic use at 2 years as compared with all other groups. In conclusion, COMB index treatment conferred an overall long-term remission advantage when medications were tapered before termination of initial CBT-I treatment, and COMB subjects were not prone to greater future hypnotic use.

A further retrospective analysis of the 2009 study data by Morin and colleagues in 2014[106] addressed further qualitative aspects of sleep diary-based changes in sleep during that first 6-week stage of treatment (**Fig. 1**). COMB substantially outperformed CBT-I during the first week of treatment regarding improvements in SOL, WASO, SE, TST preservation (ie, less decline in TST), and SQ, and this COMB advantage persisted for most treatment weeks. COMB subjects achieved maximum (100%) improvement in SOL, WASO, and SE after only 1 to 2 weeks of treatment and aftrer only 3 weeks for SQ, whereas the CBT-I group did not achieve maximum improvement until 2 weeks for SOL and 3 weeks for WASO and SE, and, significantly, CBT-I monotherapy subjects attained only 80% of their maximum SQ by the fifth treatment week, only vaulting to its zenith at the 6th and final session.. Also, most strikingly, during the first week of treatment, CBT-I subjects displayed a dramatic 16.6% reduction in their TST (average 58 min less sleep), whereas COMB subjects reduced TST by only 6% to 8% (average 24 min less sleep). Both groups gradually increased TST over the remaining 5 weeks. None of these early COMB sleep advantages seemed to predict eventual sleep outcomes as determined by the ISI. Nor did early COMB improvements seem to impact compliance. In conclusion, COMB produced a more rapid onset of improvement in sleep diary parameters than did CBT-I, a benefit advantage sustained for SQ from almost start to finish, though these COMB advantages could not be shown to impact outcomes at 6 weeks.

Morin and colleagues, 2020: This study[107] compared monotherapy switching strategies for BT non-remitters. 211 subjects, which included patients diagnosed with comorbid medical and psychiatric illnesses, were randomized to either 6 weeks of treatment with zolpidem or BT, which

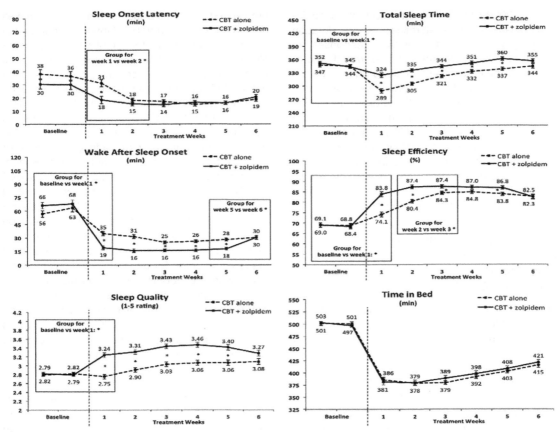

Fig. 1 Weekly sleep diary data CBT+zolpidem vs CBT .*, statistically significant. (Excerpted from Morin and colleagues, 2014.[106])

uses SRT and stimulus control (SCT), but not cognitive therapy, as core treatment components. Non-remitters to zolpidem were randomized to a second-stage treatment of either BT or trazodone, whereas BT non-remitters were randomized to the second-stage CBT-I or zolpidem. Study results demonstrated that both first-stage treatments produced equal response and remission rates, but that a second-stage treatment added significantly to overall remission rates, especially for patients with psychiatric comorbidity (these patients who remitted less to BT than did non-comorbid patients in the first stage). The largest added value remission improvement occurred for sequences beginning with BT (BT to zolpidem 38.1% to 55%, respectively). As expected, pharmacologic only treatment sequences afforded significantly greater improvement in TST than sequences involving BT or CBT-I. In conclusion, though ID patients with psychiatric comorbidity exhibited treatment resistance to BT, adding a second-stage treatment, such as zolpidem, allowed these patients to remit at rates on par with non-comorbid patients.

Edinger and colleagues, 2022: Edinger and colleagues[108] conducted a further analysis of the Morin 2020 study data, addressing pretreatment patient characteristics that moderated responses to the different treatment sequences. Baseline higher levels of fatigue, higher psychopathology defined as the presence of psychiatric comorbidity in addition to a lower than 50th percentile score on a measure of mental health self-perception (ie, negative perception), subjective short sleep duration (TST <6 hour), and low SE (<75%) were all associated with increased levels of non-remission and attrition, mostly powered by sequences starting with BT. In conclusion, it seemed that certain specific patient pretreatment characteristics predicted potential treatment resistance to BT, though such patients could attain significant benefit with a switch to a second-stage treatment, such as zolpidem.

Returning a moment to the topic of TST, Edinger's analysis of Morin's 2020 results could be interpreted as supporting the notion that short TST is a marker for CBT-I poor response. However, a retrospective analysis by Rochefort using

Morin's 2009 COMB trial data found no association between PSG-determined short duration sleep (<6 hour) and improved responses to COMB as compared with CBT-I, as would be predicted by the objective short sleep phenotype hypothesis. It should be noted, however, that objective short sleepers still attained remission 21% less often with CBT-I monotherapy than did normal sleepers (25% vs 46% respectively). In conclusion, Rochefort's analysis, the only one to address differential responses in objective short sleepers based on data derived from an actual COMB RCT, did not confirm that COMB offers an advantage for objective short sleepers.[109]

APPLICATION OF RANDOMIZED CONTROLLED TRIAL FINDINGS AND DISCUSSION
Short-Term Outcomes

The RCT findings, particularly Morin and colleagues' 2009 study, confirm some core theoretical assumptions based on monotherapy research. First, COMB and CBT-I confer about equal remission rates by the end of an index 6-week treatment course. Second, COMB did not seem to confer harm by either interfering with CBT-I-related outcomes or increasing the risk for serious adverse consequences, including PCT dependence, misuse, and abuse. Third, though observational, COMB patients appeared to, rather than overusing zolpidem, to underuse it during the acute treatment period (less than 100% compliance with taking the required amount of zolpidem, falling further to <80% in the last week of treatment). Even during the less structured 6-month extended treatment period, COMB patients allowed as-needed zolpidem only tended to use one-half of their 10 pill per month allotment.

Where COMB seems to offer a substantial advantage versus CBT-I monotherapy is in regard to trajectory of sleep diary-reported benefit. Based on the Morin 2014 retrospective analysis of the 2009 trial data,[106] COMB subjects improved on all sleep parameters (SOL, SE, WASO, and SQ) at week 1 and experienced a markedly attenuated rate of decline in TST compared with CBT-I monotherapy subjects. The ability of COMB to soften this precipitous drop in TST in the early weeks was extraordinary. CBT-I monotherapy subjects lost an average of 16.6% of their baseline TST, or 58 minutes less sleep, whereas the COMB average loss was 6.8%, or 24 minutes less sleep. SQ for CBT-I subjects barely catches up to that for COMB even at the last (sixth) week of treatment. The fact that

time in bed (TIB) was equal for both groups makes such a result more notable. Observationally, early significant superiority for COMB in blunting the slope of TST decline and preserving SE, as compared with CBT-I, occurs concurrently with the COMB patient's perception of better sleep (SQ), especially in the first 1 or 2 weeks. This SQ advantage for COMB persists throughout the treatment. However, linkage of this considerable early COMB benefit with reduced attrition or increased compliance could not be established. Attrition was no different overall between COMB and CBT-I groups. Here, it may be worth noting that RCTs involving CBT-I or SRT as stand-alone treatments, demonstrate very low attrition rates, around 8%, which is comparable to controls.[24] Such results are significantly better than the rates reported for general sleep clinic populations, where dropouts can be as high as 40%, even for face-to-face treated CBT-I patients before the fourth week of treatment.[25] As might be expected, unidentified RCT-related factors likely mitigate against attrition, even for patients who are more vulnerable to dropping out in a less structured setting. For such patients in real-world settings, perceived earlier improvement in sleep may be the key element that prevents treatment discontinuation and allows the patient to persevere with CBT-I. Importantly, it must be emphasized that no COMB RCT has specifically addressed CBT-I treatment-resistant patients. Morin 2020, though not technically a COMB study, may provide some help as it addresses treatment resistance, though to BT, not CBT-I. BT shares with CBT-I employment of SRT and SCT as treatment components, so perhaps some cross assumptions can be allowed. Patients not remitting to BT received a significant boost in remission when provided a second-stage treatment such as zolpidem. Perhaps this study should reasonably be viewed as a COMB study. As CBT-I and BT are both learned paradigms, an imprint is left, like a gift that keeps giving. Such treatments likely alter perceptions, even for non-remitters. Zolpidem may be acting essentially as an add-on for patients who have achieved some benefit from BT, though not enough to cross the remission threshold (being mindful that no treatment controls were present in this study). Zolpidem provided prior to BT treatment termination could, just as well, confer rescue for these more resistant patients, perhaps even staving off non-remission. In conclusion, by merging the findings from Morin 2009 and Morin 2020, it becomes possible to visualize that COMB could indeed assist certain CBT-I (or BT) treatment-resistant patients in achieving remission. Future trials enriched with

CBT-I treatment-resistant patients could attain sufficienting power capable of reveiling that COMB early benefits do translate to improved index treatment outcomes for this group.

Long-Term Outcomes

As noted, an acute course of COMB did not signal any interference with longer term maintenance of remission compared with subjects receiving CBT-I monotherapy. In fact, the pooled results of Morin 2009 for all stage 1 COMB patients were indicative of increased remission rates after 6 months of extended treatment and again 6 months after that (1 year post-index 6-week treatment). As well, COMB patients did not engage in greater prescription hypnotic use at 2 years compared with CBT-I monotherapy patients. Long-term benefits were best maintained with COMB when PCT was tapered before index treatment termination. It may be that CBT-I conferred self-efficacy acquisition,[14,76] postulated to provide an essential underpinning for CBT-I's posttreatment durable benefit, is not undermined by the time-limited use of PCT early in treatment.

COMB Predictors, Moderators, and Mediators of Benefit

RCT findings, especially Morin's 2014 examination of the 2009 data, demonstrate that COMB at first outperforms CBT-I during the early phases of treatment, an advantage potentially mediated by perceived sleep improvement. Such data correlate with research reporting that most patients who drop out when receiving CBT-I do so before the fourth week of treatment. Those first 4 weeks are a high-risk period for patients and may serve as an optimal time to initiate COMB. COMB is capable of providing subjective gains that can help compensate for the short-term pain.

How COMB improves a patient's perception that they are obtaining better SQ is left unresolved. COMB quickly blunts the SRT-induced slide in TST along with improving SE. Both short duration sleep and sleep continuity disturbance (as reflected by SE) have been shown to be independent risk factors for CBT-I intolerance and attrition.[108] The data derived from Morin 2009 support that zolpidem can help preserve TST while also increasing SE during these tenuous first weeks of SRT. As discussed above, neurobiological sleep research suggests that BZRAs can quickly enhance GABAergic control over upregulated arousal intrusion, strengthening the NREM/REM flip flop switch.[89,95] COMB may band-aid these microstructural wounds temporarily until SRT finishes

its job and CBT-I can go it alone, getting all the credit.

Clinically, there is little a practitioner can do to detect the ID endotype that directs a treatment decision toward COMB. Despite Rochefort's conclusion that COMB did not moderate outcomes based on pretreatment sleep duration in the Morin 2009 study, ISSD patients still remitted with CBT-I monotherapy less often than normal sleepers. For now, more basic but clinically relevant indicators of sleep improvement, such as patient-reported SQ, should be kept in the clinician's sites. Better sleep diary SQ scores pre- and post-CBT-I treatment sessions are reported to be conducive to improved adherence.[101] Some patients may need to experience that "good night's sleep" sooner than others to stay on board with CBT-I. Conversely, it may be that intractable low SQ scores pre- and post-CBT-I session could serve as a clinical marker for prompting early clinician direct inquiry with the patient as to how they are feeling about treatment and their progress. Although there is no specific objective clinical measure that reflects disillusionment, the clinician may be best able to detect that this is occurring by virtue of a personal interaction. At such a point, the offering up of additional clinical options, including in a manner that of COMB, within a discourse that respects patient preference[120], can allow for a mutually agreed decision as to how to move forward that can reenergize the therapeutic alliance and potentially head off patient attrition.

CLINICAL CARE POINTS AND TREATMENT SUGGESTIONS

Although the following suggestions are largely based on RCT findings, they should not be construed as approximating truly evidence-based recommendations. Though some are consistent with presently supported standards of treatment (such as #1), others are highly speculative in nature and require significant further investigation (such as #7, 8, and 9).

1. Full-component CBT-I monotherapy should be advocated as the initial treatment of choice for almost all ID patients, exceptions being SRT contraindicated comorbid disorders such as comorbid bipolar I disorder and epilepsy. Owing to the infrequent but potentially serious risks conferred by PCT, COMB should generally not be promoted as an initial option for patients considering CBT-I treatment.
2. COMB should be offered as an adaptive alternative for patients engaging in CBT-I monotherapy who appear to be progressing poorly and

at risk for not completing adequately a full course of treatment.

3. COMB may be most effective when initiated early during the course of CBT-I, within the first 4 weeks, a key period for increased risk of treatment attrition.

4. Taper and discontinuation of PCT should be completed before CBT-I termination. Taper of a BZRA can occur quickly, allowing for remaining treatment sessions that consist only of CBT-I, devoid of adjunctive PCT, perhaps producing better long term outcomes by allowing patients to connect their ongoing progress to CBT-I and not medication.

5. When offering COMB, the risks and benefits of PCT should be addressed fully with the patient, including a clear communication that although PCT can confer certain serious side effects and induce dependency, PCT can also provide an established rapid improvement in sleep quality. An offer of COMB should only occur after a comprehensive medical evaluation that assesses modifiable and non-modifiable risk factors for PCT-conferred adverse events.

6. Pretreatment patient characteristics such as short TST, low SE, higher psychopathology, and objective sleep duration phenotype, should not be relied on for COMB treatment decisions but can serve to heighten clinician awareness to the potential for CBT-I non-remission.

7. Within-treatment indicators of responsiveness to CBT-I should serve as the most preeminent factors triggering an offer of COMB. Low SQ scores on sleep diary that fail to improve or continue to decline, especially proximal to CBT-I sessions, should serve as a prompt for direct inquiry with the patient regarding treatment attitudes, distress, disillusionment, and motivation to continue with treatment. Higher SQ scores in close proximity to CBT-I sessions have been associated with improved adherence to CBT-I. COMB can rapidly improve SQ scores.

8. COMB rescue can also be offered later in treatment, when patients appear unlikely to remit. PCT taper can be reattempted along with provision of extended CBT-I sessions, a likely low-harm approach.

9. COMB RCT evidence exists almost solely for zolpidem. Results suggest zolpidem add-on to CBT-I confers low harm and noninterference with longer term outcomes when compared with CBT-I monotherapy. As such, intermediate half-life, such as zolpidem and eszopiclone, BZRAs can serve as appropriate initial choices for COMB purposes unless contraindications exist (ie, history of CSRBs or active SUD).

CAVEATS AND THE FUTURE

The suggestions offered in this narrative review will require further research involving larger subject populations that include more treatment-resistant patients. Actigraphy shows some promise as a low-burden approach that can serve as an appropriate adjunct to sleep diary reports, providing some objective pretreatment and within-treatment indicators of sleep fragmentation or discrepancy between subjective reports and objective results.[29] Such actigraphy data may help direct whether a patient should not receive hypnotics, such as in insufficient sleep syndrome[121], or perhaps paradoxical insomnia[29]. In addition, hypnotics that act by inhibiting arousal via mechanisms different from that of BZRAs, such as anti-orexigenic DORAs, deserve inclusion in future COMB studies. Finally, controversy continues over whether a subset of hyper-aroused medically at-risk ID patients would do better with continuous PCT after an acute course of CBT-I, a debate that will not be settled soon.

SUMMARY

COMB, using an intermediate half-life BZRA such as zolpidem, seems to be an effective and low-harm adaptation to CBT-I that can provide a more rapid trajectory of improvement in perceived sleep quality without interfering with the long-lasting posttreatment benefit that can occur with CBT-I monotherapy. Owing to the potential risks conferred by PCT, COMB is best directed toward patients responding poorly to CBT-I and judged to be at risk for non-remission. After appropriate risk–benefit determination, COMB can be an appropriate adaptation that should immediately improve a patient's sleep quality, potentially enhancing adherence and ultimately preserving the opportunity for a CBT-I associated remission for at-risk patients.

DISCLOSURE

The authors have nothing to disclose.

REFERENCES

1. Morin CM, Vallières A, Guay B, et al. Cognitive behavioral therapy, singly and combined with medication, for persistent insomnia: a randomized controlled trial. JAMA 2009;301(19):2005–15.

2. Buysse DJ. Chronic insomnia. Am J Psychiatry 2008;165(6):678–86.

3. Sivertsen B, Pallesen S, Glozier N, et al. Midlife insomnia and subsequent mortality: the Hordaland health study. BMC public health 2014;14(1):1–10.

4. Shahly V, Berglund PA, Coulouvrat C, et al. The associations of insomnia with costly workplace accidents and errors: results from the America Insomnia Survey. Arch Gen Psychiatry 2012; 69(10):1054–63.

5. Laugsand LE, Strand LB, Vatten LJ, et al. Insomnia symptoms and risk for unintentional fatal injuries—the HUNT study. Sleep 2014;37(11):1777–86.

6. Sivertsen B, Krokstad S, Øverland S, et al. The epidemiology of insomnia: associations with physical and mental health.: the HUNT-2 study. J psychosomatic Res 2009;67(2):109–16.

7. Riemann D, Perlis ML. The treatments of chronic insomnia: a review of benzodiazepine receptor agonists and psychological and behavioral therapies. Sleep Med Rev 2009;13(3):205–14.

8. Fernandez-Mendoza J, Vgontzas AN, Liao D, et al. Insomnia with objective short sleep duration and incident hypertension: the Penn State Cohort. Hypertension 2012;60(4):929–35.

9. Vgontzas AN, Fernandez-Mendoza J, Liao D, et al. Insomnia with objective short sleep duration: the most biologically severe phenotype of the disorder. Sleep Med Rev 2013;17(4):241–54.

10. Sateia MJ, Buysse DJ, Krystal AD, et al. Clinical practice guideline for the pharmacologic treatment of chronic insomnia in adults: an American Academy of Sleep Medicine clinical practice guideline. J Clin Sleep Med 2017;13(2):307–49.

11. Schutte-Rodin S, Broch L, Buysse D, et al. Clinical guideline for the evaluation and management of chronic insomnia in adults. J Clin Sleep Med 2008;4(5):487–504.

12. Edinger JD, Arnedt JT, Bertisch SM, et al. Behavioral and psychological treatments for chronic insomnia disorder in adults: an American Academy of Sleep Medicine clinical practice guideline. J Clin Sleep Med 2021;17(2):255–62.

13. Morin CM, Belleville G, Bélanger L, et al. The Insomnia Severity Index: psychometric indicators to detect insomnia cases and evaluate treatment response. Sleep 2011;34(5):601–8.

14. Wu R, Bao J, Zhang C, et al. Comparison of sleep condition and sleep-related psychological activity after cognitive-behavior and pharmacological therapy for chronic insomnia. Psychother Psychosom 2006;75(4):220–8.

15. Cheung JM, Ji X-W, Morin CM. Cognitive behavioral therapies for insomnia and hypnotic medications: considerations and controversies. Sleep Med Clin 2019;14(2):253–65.

16. Harbourt K, Nevo ON, Zhang R, et al. Association of eszopiclone, zaleplon, or zolpidem with complex sleep behaviors resulting in serious injuries, including death. Pharmacoepidemiol Drug Saf 2020;29(6):684–91.

17. Morin CM, Altena E, Ivers H, et al. Insomnia, hypnotic use, and road collisions: a population-based, 5-year cohort study. Sleep 2020;43(8):zsaa032.

18. Baglioni C, Bostanova Z, Bacaro V, et al. A systematic review and network meta-analysis of randomized controlled trials evaluating the evidence base of melatonin, light exposure, exercise, and complementary and alternative medicine for patients with insomnia disorder. J Clin Med 2020; 9(6):1949.

19. Avidan AY, Fries BE, James ML, et al. Insomnia and hypnotic use, recorded in the minimum data set, as predictors of falls and hip fractures in Michigan nursing homes. J Am Geriatr Soc 2005;53(6): 955–62.

20. Morin CM, Colecchi C, Stone J, et al. Behavioral and pharmacological therapies for late-life insomnia: a randomized controlled trial. JAMA 1999;281(11):991–9.

21. Kyle SD, Miller CB, Rogers Z, et al. Sleep restriction therapy for insomnia is associated with reduced objective total sleep time, increased daytime somnolence, and objectively impaired vigilance: implications for the clinical management of insomnia disorder. Sleep 2014;37(2):229–37.

22. Kyle SD, Morgan K, Spiegelhalder K, et al. No pain, no gain: an exploratory within-subjects mixed-methods evaluation of the patient experience of sleep restriction therapy (SRT) for insomnia. Sleep Med 2011;12(8):735–47.

23. Miller CB, Espie CA, Bartlett DJ, et al. Acceptability, tolerability, and potential efficacy of cognitive behavioural therapy for insomnia disorder subtypes defined by polysomnography: a retrospective cohort study. Scientific Rep 2018;8(1): 1–6.

24. Maurer LF, Schneider J, Miller CB, et al. The clinical effects of sleep restriction therapy for insomnia: a meta-analysis of randomised controlled trials. Sleep Med Rev 2021;58:101493.

25. Ong JC, Kuo TF, Manber R. Who is at risk for dropout from group cognitive-behavior therapy for insomnia? J psychosomatic Res 2008;64(4): 419–25.

26. Morin CM, Jarrin DC, Ivers H, et al. Incidence, persistence, and remission rates of insomnia over 5 years. JAMA Netw open 2020;3(11):e2018782.

27. Morin CM, Bélanger L, Bastien C, et al. Long-term outcome after discontinuation of benzodiazepines for insomnia: a survival analysis of relapse. Behav Res Ther 2005;43(1):1–14.

28. Morin CM. Combined therapeutics for insomnia: should our first approach be behavioral or pharmacological? Sleep Med 2006;7:S15–9 [published Online First: Epub Date]].

29. Fernandez-Mendoza J. CBT-I in the short sleep duration phenotype. United Kingdom: Adapting

Cognitive Behavioral Therapy for Insomnia: Elsevier; 2022. p. 369–401.

30. Davidson JR, Dickson C, Han H. Cognitive behavioural treatment for insomnia in primary care: a systematic review of sleep outcomes. Br J Gen Pract 2019;69(686):e657–64.

31. Benz F, Knoop T, Ballesio A, et al. The efficacy of cognitive and behavior therapies for insomnia on daytime symptoms: a systematic review and network meta-analysis. Clin Psychol Rev 2020;80: 101873.

32. Omvik S, Sivertsen B, Pallesen S, et al. Daytime functioning in older patients suffering from chronic insomnia: treatment outcome in a randomized controlled trial comparing CBT with zopiclone. Behav Res Ther 2008;46(5):623–41.

33. Fava M, McCall WV, Krystal A, et al. Eszopiclone co-administered with fluoxetine in patients with insomnia coexisting with major depressive disorder. Biol Psychiatry 2006;59(11):1052–60.

34. Pollack MH, Van Ameringen M, Simon NM, et al. A double-blind randomized controlled trial of augmentation and switch strategies for refractory social anxiety disorder. Am J Psychiatry 2014; 171(1):44–53.

35. Pollack MH, Hoge EA, Worthington JJ, et al. Eszopiclone for the treatment of posttraumatic stress disorder and associated insomnia: a randomized, double-blind, placebo-controlled trial. J Clin Psychiatry 2011;72(7):6681.

36. Trockel M, Karlin BE, Taylor CB, et al. Effects of cognitive behavioral therapy for insomnia on suicidal ideation in veterans. Sleep 2015;38(2): 259–65.

37. Christensen H, Batterham PJ, Gosling JA, et al. Effectiveness of an online insomnia program (SHUTi) for prevention of depressive episodes (the GoodNight Study): a randomised controlled trial. Lancet Psychiatry 2016;3(4):333–41.

38. Baglioni C, Battagliese G, Feige B, et al. Insomnia as a predictor of depression: a meta-analytic evaluation of longitudinal epidemiological studies. J Affective Disord 2011;135:10–9.

39. Wang Y-Y, Yang Y, Rao W-W, et al. Cognitive behavioural therapy monotherapy for insomnia: a meta-analysis of randomized controlled trials. Asian J Psychiatry 2020;49:101828.

40. Mason M, Cates CJ, Smith I. Effects of opioid, hypnotic and sedating medications on sleep-disordered breathing in adults with obstructive sleep apnoea. Cochrane Database Syst Rev 2015;7:1–57.

41. Manber R, Buysse DJ, Edinger J, et al. Efficacy of cognitive-behavioral therapy for insomnia combined with antidepressant pharmacotherapy in patients with comorbid depression and insomnia: a randomized controlled trial. J Clin Psychiatry 2016;77(10):2446.

42. Wu JQ, Appleman ER, Salazar RD, et al. Cognitive behavioral therapy for insomnia comorbid with psychiatric and medical conditions: a meta-analysis. JAMA Intern Med 2015;175(9):1461–72.

43. Irwin MR, Carrillo C, Sadeghi N, et al. Prevention of incident and recurrent major depression in older adults with insomnia: a randomized clinical trial. JAMA Psychiatry 2022;79(1):33–41.

44. Cassidy-Eagle EL, Siebern A, Chen H, et al. Cognitive-behavioral therapy for insomnia in older adults. Cogn Behav Pract 2021;29(1):146–60.

45. Simpson N, Manber R. CBT-I in patients who wish to reduce use of hypnotic medication. United Kingdom: Adapting Cognitive Behavioral Therapy for Insomnia: Elsevier; 2022. p. 437–56.

46. Takaesu Y, Utsumi T, Okajima I, et al. Psychosocial intervention for discontinuing benzodiazepine hypnotics in patients with chronic insomnia: a systematic review and meta-analysis. Sleep Med Rev 2019;48:101214.

47. Morin CM, Bastien C, Guay B, et al. Randomized clinical trial of supervised tapering and cognitive behavior therapy to facilitate benzodiazepine discontinuation in older adults with chronic insomnia. Am J Psychiatry 2004;161(2):332–42.

48. Nowakowski S, Garland S, Grandner MA, et al. Adapting cognitive behavioral therapy for insomnia. United Kingdom: Elsevier; 2021.

49. Oroz R, Kung S, Croarkin PE, et al. Transcranial magnetic stimulation therapeutic applications on sleep and insomnia: a review. Sleep Sci Pract 2021;5(1):1–10.

50. Chamine I, Atchley R, Oken BS. Hypnosis intervention effects on sleep outcomes: a systematic review. J Clin Sleep Med 2018;14(2):271–83.

51. Richter K, Myllymaeki J, Scharold-Schaefer S, et al. Treating comorbid insomnia in older adults via cognitive-behavioural treatment, bright light and exercise. Health 2014;2014:960–8.

52. Nutt DJ, Stahl SM. Searching for perfect sleep: the continuing evolution of GABAA receptor modulators as hypnotics. J Psychopharmacol 2010; 24(11):1601–12.

53. Greenblatt DJ, Harmatz JS, Roth T. Zolpidem and gender: are women really at risk? J Clin Psychopharmacol 2019;39(3):189–99.

54. Neubauer DN. Insomnia pharmacotherapies: pharmacodynamics, strategies, new directions, and key measures in clinical trials. Handbook Behav Neurosci 2019;30:639–48.

55. Huedo-Medina TB, Kirsch I, Middlemass J, et al. Effectiveness of non-benzodiazepine hypnotics in treatment of adult insomnia: meta-analysis of data submitted to the Food and Drug Administration. BMJ 2012;345:1–13.

56. Perlis ML, McCall WV, Krystal AD, et al. Long-term, non-nightly administration of zolpidem in the

treatment of patients with primary insomnia. J Clin Psychiatry 2004;65(8):10719.

57. Hockenhull J, Black JC, Haynes CM, et al. Nonmedical use of benzodiazepines and Z-drugs in the UK. Br J Clin Pharmacol 2021;87(4): 1676–83.

58. Votaw VR, Geyer R, Rieselbach MM, et al. The epidemiology of benzodiazepine misuse: a systematic review. Drug and alcohol dependence 2019;200:95–114.

59. Stahl SM. Stahl's essential psychopharmacology: neuroscientific basis and practical applications. Cambridge university press; 2021.

60. Roehrs TA, Randall S, Harris E, et al. Twelve months of nightly zolpidem does not lead to rebound insomnia or withdrawal symptoms: a prospective placebo-controlled study. J Psychopharmacol 2012;26(8):1088–95.

61. Ji X, Ivers H, Savard J, et al. Residual symptoms after natural remission of insomnia: associations with relapse over 4 years. Sleep 2019;42(8):zsz122.

62. Perrier J, Bertran F, Marie S, et al. Impaired driving performance associated with effect of time duration in patients with primary insomnia. Sleep 2014;37(9):1565–73.

63. Leger D, Bayon V, Ohayon MM, et al. Insomnia and accidents: cross-sectional study (EQUINOX) on sleep-related home, work and car accidents in 5293 subjects with insomnia from 10 countries. J Sleep Res 2014;23(2):143–52.

64. Hägg SA, Torén K, Lindberg E. Role of sleep disturbances in occupational accidents among women. Scand J Work Environ Health 2015;41(4):368–76.

65. Wardle-Pinkston S, Slavish DC, Taylor DJ. Insomnia and cognitive performance: a systematic review and meta-analysis. Sleep Med Rev 2019;48:101205.

66. Drake CL, Vargas I, Roth T, et al. Quantitative measures of nocturnal insomnia symptoms predict greater deficits across multiple daytime impairment domains. Behav Sleep Med 2015;13(1):73–87.

67. Chen T-Y, Lee S, Buxton OM. A greater extent of insomnia symptoms and physician-recommended sleep medication use predict fall risk in community-dwelling older adults. Sleep 2017; 40(11):zsx142.

68. Rumble ME, McCall WV, Dickson DA, et al. An exploratory analysis of the association of circadian rhythm dysregulation and insomnia with suicidal ideation over the course of treatment in individuals with depression, insomnia, and suicidal ideation. J Clin Sleep Med 2020;16(8):1311–9.

69. Dawson D, Sprajcer M, Thomas M. How much sleep do you need? A comprehensive review of fatigue related impairment and the capacity to work or drive safely. Accid Anal Prev 2021;151: 105955.

70. Lian Y, Xiao J, Liu Y, et al. Associations between insomnia, sleep duration and poor work ability. J psychosomatic Res 2015;78(1):45–51.

71. Walsh JK, Krystal AD, Amato DA, et al. Nightly treatment of primary insomnia with eszopiclone for six months: effect on sleep, quality of life, and work limitations. Sleep 2007;30(8):959–68.

72. Roehrs TA, Roth T. Hyperarousal in insomnia and hypnotic dose escalation. Sleep Med 2016;23: 16–20.

73. Halli-Tierney A, Scarbrough C, Carroll DG. Polypharmacy: evaluating risks and deprescribing. Am Fam Physician 2019;100(1):32–8.

74. Guina J, Merrill B. Benzodiazepines I: upping the care on downers: the evidence of risks, benefits and alternatives. J Clin Med 2018;7(2):17.

75. Melani MS, Paiva JM, Silva MC, et al. Absence of definitive scientific evidence that benzodiazepines could hinder the efficacy of exposure-based interventions in adults with anxiety or posttraumatic stress disorders: a systematic review of randomized clinical trials. Depress Anxiety 2020;37(12): 1231–42.

76. Parsons CE, Zachariae R, Landberger C, et al. How does cognitive behavioural therapy for insomnia work? A systematic review and meta-analysis of mediators of change. Clin Psychol Rev 2021;86:102027.

77. Cho JH, Kremer S, Young J. Who to refer to a behavioral insomnia clinic?—recommendations based on treatment rationale and response prediction. Curr Sleep Med Rep 2021;7(4):1–8.

78. Matthews EE, Schmiege SJ, Cook PF, et al. Adherence to cognitive behavioral therapy for insomnia (CBTI) among women following primary breast cancer treatment: a pilot study. Behav Sleep Med 2012;10(3):217–29.

79. Perlis ML, Pigeon WR, Grandner MA, et al. Why treat insomnia? J Prim Care Community Health 2021;12. 21501327211014084.

80. Smith MT, Perlis ML, Park A, et al. Comparative meta-analysis of pharmacotherapy and behavior therapy for persistent insomnia. Am J Psychiatry 2002;159(1):5–11.

81. Vgontzas AN, Puzino K, Fernandez-Mendoza J, et al. Effects of trazodone versus cognitive behavioral therapy in the insomnia with short sleep duration phenotype: a preliminary study. J Clin Sleep Med 2020;16(12):2009–19.

82. Bathgate CJ, Edinger JD, Krystal AD. Insomnia patients with objective short sleep duration have a blunted response to cognitive behavioral therapy for insomnia. Sleep 2017;40(1):zsw012.

83. Galbiati A, Sforza M, Fasiello E, et al. Impact of phenotypic heterogeneity of insomnia on the patients' response to cognitive-behavioral therapy

for insomnia: current perspectives. Nat Sci Sleep 2019;11:367.

84. Plante DT. The evolving nexus of sleep and depression. Am J Psychiatry 2021;178(10):896–902.

85. McCall WV, Benca RM, Rosenquist PB, et al. Reducing suicidal ideation through insomnia treatment (REST-IT): a randomized clinical trial. Am J Psychiatry 2019;176(11):957–65.

86. Trockel M, Karlin BE, Taylor CB, et al. Cognitive behavioral therapy for insomnia with veterans: evaluation of effectiveness and correlates of treatment outcomes. Behav Res Ther 2014;53:41–6.

87.. Guzman SG. Cognitive behavioral therapy to support sleep for psychiatric patients with insomnia. Ann Arbour, MI: ProqQuest; 2020.

88. Mason BL, Davidov A, Minhajuddin A, et al. Focusing on insomnia symptoms to better understand depression: a STAR* D report. J affective Disord 2020;260:183–6.

89. Riemann D, Krone LB, Wulff K, et al. Sleep, insomnia, and depression. Neuropsychopharmacology 2020;45(1):74–89.

90. Spielman AJ, Yang C-M, Glovinsky PB. Sleep restriction therapy. Behavioral treatments for sleep disorders. Elsevier; 2011. p. 9–19.

91. Becker SP, Tamm L, Epstein JN, et al. Impact of sleep restriction on affective functioning in adolescents with attention-deficit/hyperactivity disorder. J Child Psychol Psychiatry 2020;61(10):1160–8.

92. Stone KL, Blackwell TL, Ancoli-Israel S, et al. Sleep disturbances and risk of falls in older community-dwelling men: the outcomes of Sleep Disorders in Older Men (MrOS Sleep) Study. J Am Geriatr Soc 2014;62(2):299–305.

93. Stone KL, Ancoli-Israel S, Blackwell T, et al. Actigraphy-measured sleep characteristics and risk of falls in older women. Arch Intern Med 2008;168(16):1768–75.

94. Stone KL, Ewing SK, Lui LY, et al. Self-reported sleep and nap habits and risk of falls and fractures in older women: the study of osteoporotic fractures. J Am Geriatr Soc 2006;54(8):1177–83.

95. Kim JJ, Hibbs RE. Direct structural insights into GABAA receptor pharmacology. Trends Biochem Sci 2021;46(6):502–17.

96. Wilkerson A, Boals A, Taylor DJ. Sharpening our understanding of the consequences of insomnia: the relationship between insomnia and everyday cognitive failures. Cogn Ther Res 2012;36(2):134–9.

97. Quadri S, Drake C, Hudgel DW. Improvement of idiopathic central sleep apnea with zolpidem. J Clin Sleep Med 2009;5(2):122–9.

98. Eckert DJ, Sweetman A. Impaired central control of sleep depth propensity as a common mechanism for excessive overnight wake time: implications

for sleep apnea, insomnia and beyond. J Clin Sleep Med 2020;16(3):341–3.

99. Wang D, Tang Y, Chen Y, et al. The effect of non-benzodiazepine sedative hypnotics on CPAP adherence in patients with OSA: a systematic review and meta-analysis. Sleep 2021;44(8): zsab077.

100. Lin BM, Hu FB, Curhan GC. Association between benzodiazepine receptor agonists and snoring among women in the nurses' health study. JAMA Otolaryngology–Head Neck Surg 2017;143(2): 162–7.

101. Mellor A, Kavaliotis E, Mascaro L, et al. Approaches to the assessment of adherence to CBT-I, predictors of adherence, and the association of adherence to outcomes: a systematic review. Sleep Med Rev 2022;63:101620.

102. Van Someren EJ. Brain mechanisms of insomnia: new perspectives on causes and consequences. Physiol Rev 2021;101(3):995–1046.

103. Jacobs GD, Pace-Schott EF, Stickgold R, et al. Cognitive behavior therapy and pharmacotherapy for insomnia: a randomized controlled trial and direct comparison. Arch Intern Med 2004;164(17): 1888–96.

104. Vallières A, Morin CM, Guay B. Sequential combinations of drug and cognitive behavioral therapy for chronic insomnia: an exploratory study. Behav Res Ther 2005;43(12):1611–30.

105. Beaulieu-Bonneau S, Ivers H, Guay B, et al. Long-term maintenance of therapeutic gains associated with cognitive-behavioral therapy for insomnia delivered alone or combined with zolpidem. Sleep 2017;40(3). https://doi.org/10.1093/sleep/zsx002.

106. Morin CM, Beaulieu-Bonneau S, Ivers H, et al. Speed and trajectory of changes of insomnia symptoms during acute treatment with cognitive–behavioral therapy, singly and combined with medication. Sleep Med 2014;15(6):701–7.

107. Morin CM, Edinger JD, Beaulieu-Bonneau S, et al. Effectiveness of sequential psychological and medication therapies for insomnia disorder: a randomized clinical trial. JAMA psychiatry 2020; 77(11):1107–15.

108. Edinger JD, Beaulieu-Bonneau S, Ivers H, et al. Association between insomnia patients' pre-treatment characteristics and their responses to distinctive treatment sequences. Sleep 2022;45(1):zsab245.

109. Rochefort A, Jarrin DC, Bélanger L, et al. Insomnia treatment response as a function of objectively measured sleep duration. Sleep Med 2019;56: 135–44.

110. Perlis M, McCall W, Krystal A, et al. Long-term, non-nightly administration of zolpidem in the treatment of patients with primary insomnia. J Clin Psychiatry 2004;65(8):1128–37.

111. Kay D, Buysse D. Hyperarousal and beyond: new insights to the pathophysiology of insomnia disorder through functional neuroimaging studies. Brain Sci 2017;7(3):23.

112. Carter S, Carberry J, Cho G, et al. Effect of 1 month of zopiclone on obstructive sleep apnoea severity and symptoms: a randomised controlled trial. Eur Respir J 2018;52(1):1–12.

113. Mir S, Wong J, Ryan C, et al. Concomitant benzodiazepine and opioids decrease sleep apnoea risk in chronic pain patients. ERJ Open Res 2020; 6(3):1–10.

114. Kalmbach D, Cuamatzi-Castelan A, Tonnu C, et al. Hyperarousal and sleep reactivity in insomnia: current insights. Nat Sci Sleep 2018;10:193.

115. Pillai V, Cheng P, Kalmbach D, et al. Prevalence and predictors of prescription sleep aid use among individuals with DSM-5 insomnia: the role of hyperarousal. Sleep 2016;39(4):825–32.

116. Eckert D, Sweetman A. Impaired central control of sleep depth propensity as a common mechanism for excessive overnight wake time: implications for sleep apnea, insomnia and beyond. J Clin Sleep Med 2020;16(3):341–3.

117. Cervena K, Dauvilliers Y, Espa F, et al. Effect of cognitive behavioural therapy for insomnia on sleep architecture and sleep EEG power spectra in psychophysiological insomnia. J Sleep Res 2004;13(4):385–93.

118. Schonmann Y, Goren O, Bareket R, et al. Chronic hypnotic use at 10 years—does the brand matter? Eur J Clin Pharmacol 2018;74(12):1623–31.

119. Perlis M, Smith M, Orff H, et al. The effects of modafinil and cognitive behavior therapy on sleep continuity in patients with primary insomnia. Sleep 2004;27(4):715–25.

120. Delevry D, Le Q. Effect of treatment preference in randomized controlled trials: systematic review of the literature and meta-analysis. Patient 2019; 12(6):593–609.

121. Smith M, McCrae C, Martin J, et al. Use of actigraphy for the evaluation of sleep disorders and circadian rhythm sleep-wake disorders: an American Academy of Sleep Medicine clinical practice guideline. J Clin Sleep Med 2018;14(7):1231–7.

Acupuncture as an Adjunct Treatment to Cognitive-Behavioral Therapy for Insomnia

Samlau Kutana, BA[a], Jun J. Mao, MD, MSCE[b], Sheila.N. Garland, PhD[a,c],*

KEYWORDS

• Insomnia • Acupuncture • Cognitive-behavioral therapy • CBT-I • Needling

KEY POINTS

- Although cognitive-behavioral therapy for insomnia (CBT-I) is recommended as a first-line treatment of insomnia, it is not equally effective in all patients.
- Acupuncture can produce clinically important improvements in insomnia severity, particularly those with objective short sleep duration and comorbid pain.
- Acupuncture is a promising adjunct treatment to CBT-I for its ability to address sleep interfering symptoms that are not targeted by CBT-I, and its low level of required engagement.

BACKGROUND

Cognitive-behavioral therapy for insomnia (CBT-I) is a manualized, multicomponent intervention recommended by the American College of Physicians and the American Academy of Sleep Medicine as the initial treatment of choice for adults presenting with insomnia disorder.[1,2] Despite the large empirical evidence base and increasing clinical adoption of CBT-I, the treatment has notable shortcomings. First, the effectiveness of CBT-I is limited by poor adherence, as many individuals struggle to implement the behavioral change strategies that are central to its efficacy.[3,4] A second concern with CBT-I is attrition, with early withdrawal rates reaching close to 40% in some studies.[5] Moreover, psychological comorbidities such as depression and anxiety that commonly present alongside insomnia have been identified as predictors of both poor adherence and early withdrawal.[4,5] Lastly, with regard to those who do not drop out

of CBT-I treatment, remission rates range from 22% to 73% and are lower in populations with comorbidities[6–9] A meta-analysis of 22 clinical trials involving 539 patients completing CBT-I found that only 36.0% reached insomnia remission status.[9] Taken together, these findings suggest that there is a sizable subgroup of patients who are unlikely to receive the full benefit from CBT-I, leaving the door open for alternative or adjunct treatment modes to address gaps in care.

In practice, insomnia presentation is often complicated by the presence of comorbidities. These commonly include psychological conditions such as anxiety, depression, as well as medical conditions such as chronic pain and vasomotor symptoms in menopausal women.[10,11] Insomnia has a complex and often bidirectional relationship with these physical and mental health conditions.[10–12] Although some studies have shown that CBT-I is able to elicit improvements in certain comorbidities such as depression, likely mediated

[a] Department of Psychology, Faculty of Science, Memorial University, 232 Elizabeth Avenue, St John's, Newfoundland A1B 3X9, Canada; [b] Department of Medicine, Memorial Sloan Kettering Cancer Center, 321 East 61st, Room 456, New York, NY 10065, USA; [c] Discipline of Oncology, Faculty of Medicine, Memorial University, 300 Prince Phillip Drive, St John's, Newfoundland A1B 3V6, Canada
* Corresponding author. Department of Psychology, Faculty of Science, Memorial University, 232 Elizabeth Avenue, St John's, Newfoundland A1B 3X9, Canada.
E-mail address: sheila.garland@mun.ca

Sleep Med Clin 18 (2023) 113–122
https://doi.org/10.1016/j.jsmc.2022.10.005
1556-407X/23/© 2022 Elsevier Inc. All rights reserved.

through improvements in insomnia, effect sizes are generally not as strong as those in treatments targeted at these symptoms directly.[8,13] Perhaps we are asking too much of CBT-I if we expect it to simultaneously address both insomnia and the whole range of conditions that are also present. For this reason, researchers and clinicians are investigating whether the addition of other evidence-based interventions can improve overall treatment response.

This review presents the rationale and support for using acupuncture as an adjunct treatment to CBT-I by (1) summarizing the evidence for using acupuncture to treat insomnia directly and indirectly through the improvement of comorbid symptoms; (2) highlighting potential challenges with implementing a combined CBT-I and acupuncture protocol including how patient characteristics and preferences differently influence response to these interventions, coordination of treatments, training requirements for dual treatment providers, access to qualified clinicians, and logistical issues such as insurance reimbursement; and (3) suggesting a future research agenda to better understand how these two interventions may work in tandem or who they may be best suited for. Being able to apply and combine effective treatments flexibly to meet the needs of the individual has the potential to reduce the burden of insomnia on the individual and society more effectively.

ACUPUNCTURE AS AN EMERGING TREATMENT OF INSOMNIA

Acupuncture, originating from traditional Chinese medicine (TCM), is a procedure in which specific body areas known as acupoints are stimulated, usually with needles (+/− electricity), to produce therapeutic effects.[14] The exact physiologic mechanisms by which acupuncture exerts its therapeutic effects are not well understood from a biomedical perspective. Growing basic research suggests that acupuncture needle stimulation can elicit changes in several neuroendocrine systems that play a role in the pathology of insomnia. Acupuncture stimulation has been shown in animal and human studies to reduce the activity of the hypothalamic-pituitary-adrenal (HPA) axis,[15] increase nocturnal melatonin release,[16] and increase levels of gamma-aminobutyric acid (GABA) while upregulating GABA-receptor expression.[15] It has also been shown to affect the sympathetic and parasympathetic axis, although research into acupuncture's effects on these systems are mixed.[15,17,18] Further, electroacupuncture at specific frequencies in animal models have shown to modulate the release of

endogenous opioids and maximize its analgesic effects,[19] which is relevant to comorbidities such as pain that present alongside insomnia. **Fig. 1** presents the proposed direct and indirect pathways by which acupuncture may exert its effects. Further research is required to clarify in which patients or conditions acupuncture impacts insomnia directly through the neuroendocrine system or indirectly by improving symptoms that are associated with insomnia (eg, pain, depression, hot flashes), or a combination of both.

Acupuncture as a Treatment of Insomnia Disorder

Trials investigating the use of acupuncture to directly treat insomnia disorder are steadily increasing. Cao and colleagues[20] reviewed 73 randomized controlled trials (RCTs) with 5,533 participants that compared any form of acupuncture (eg, manual acupuncture and electroacupuncture) with no treatment, sham acupuncture, conventional therapy, or western medications for insomnia. The pooled results on the Pittsburgh Sleep Quality Index (PSQI) showed better effect from real acupuncture than no treatment (PSQI mean difference [MD] = −5.58). Acupuncture was also found to be the more effective treatment in reducing PSQI scores when directly compared with benzodiazepine medication (PSQI MD = −1.73). Importantly, the incidence of adverse events in participants receiving benzodiazepine medications was four times larger than in participants receiving acupuncture.[20] However, only 10 of the included articles were deemed to be of high quality and poor reporting and inconsistency among included trials increased the potential risk of bias of the publications included.

Acupuncture has also been evaluated for its ability to affect objective sleep parameters. In a meta-analysis of 11 studies involving 775 patients with insomnia disorder, acupuncture was shown to increase objectively measured (eg, actigraphy, polysomnography, or micromovement-sensitive mattress/pillow sleep monitoring system) total sleep time (MD = 55 min) and sleep efficiency (MD = 9%) and reduce wake after sleep onset (MD = −6) and number of awakenings (MD = −50 min) compared with sham-/placebo acupuncture or waitlist controls.[21] In this analysis, acupuncture was also associated with a 4-point improvement on the PSQI and Insomnia Severity Index (ISI).[21] In subgroup analyses, those trials including 12 or more sessions reported better effects.[21] Still because of deficiencies in study quality, the authors rated the strength of the evidence as low to moderate, indicating that more needs

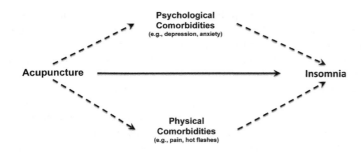

Fig. 1. Direct and indirect effects of acupuncture for insomnia.

Note: Solid line represents direct effects; Dashed lines represent indirect effects

to be done to accurately determine the effect of acupuncture on insomnia.

Acupuncture as a Treatment of Insomnia in Those with Comorbid Symptoms

In addition to exhibiting dysregulation of circadian and homeostatic sleep processes, it is not uncommon for people with insomnia disorder to have one or several comorbidities that impair sleep. These conditions range widely from back and joint pain to breast cancer, and include psychological comorbidities such as anxiety and depression, along with physiologic comorbidities such as hot flashes. Acupuncture's more general effects, mediated through both physiologic and psychological mechanisms, may confer benefit in addressing the range of sleep-impairing comorbidities.

Pain

Pain is one of the most common comorbidities that presents alongside insomnia, and is not specifically addressed by CBT-I. Pain and insomnia seem to exist in a bidirectional relationship: pain exacerbates insomnia by affecting sleep onset and maintenance, whereas sleep difficulties further increase pain sensitivity.[12,22,23] Thus, although insomnia treatment may be expected to eventually result in pain relief because of the bidirectionality of the relationship, interventions that specifically target pain may provide further, more rapid, and better sustained clinical improvements in insomnia.

Acupuncture is promising as an adjunct treatment to CBT-I in patients with pain due to its ability to address both pain and sleep simultaneously.[24] The effects of acupuncture on various types of pain have been thoroughly investigated, as pain is one of the main symptoms that acupuncture is used for in the United States.[25] Vickers and colleagues[26] are responsible for one of the largest systematic reviews of trials investigating acupuncture for four chronic pain conditions, nonspecific musculoskeletal pain, osteoarthritis, chronic headache, and shoulder pain. Results from 39 trials

involving 20,827 patients provided strong evidence that acupuncture treatment was more effective than both sham acupuncture and no acupuncture controls for each pain condition studied, providing clinically relevant pain reduction that mostly persisted (15% reduction in treatment effect) after 1 year.[26] Acupuncture's effectiveness in relieving pain has also been strongly shown in cancer populations. Reviewing the evidence from seven high-quality (sham-controlled and participant blinded) RCTs of acupuncture for cancer-related pain involving 398 participants, He and colleagues[27] found that true acupuncture was associated with reduced pain intensity compared with the sham treatment.[27] This review also found moderate evidence that acupuncture in combination with analgesic therapy was effective in helping patients reduce their opioid dosage.

Only one study to date has directly compared acupuncture to CBT-I for the treatment of insomnia in cancer survivors. This high-powered and rigorously designed RCT recruited 160 cancer survivors and randomly assigned them to acupuncture or CBT-I delivered over the course of 7 weeks. Although CBT-I was found to be more effective overall at reducing insomnia severity than acupuncture, the acupuncture group reported significantly greater improvements in comorbid pain at the end of treatment than the CBT-I group.[28] CBT-I was also significantly more effective in patients without pain at baseline.[28] These results suggest that unaddressed comorbid pain can limit CBT-I treatment response, and that acupuncture may provide further benefit to patients with moderate to severe pain. Overall, evidence supports the effectiveness of acupuncture to address issues with cancer-related pain as part of an integrated plan of care.

These findings suggest that acupuncture is effective in reducing pain of varied etiology, making it an effective non-pharmacological adjunct to CBT-I in insomnia patients with significant comorbid pain.

Depression

Patients with comorbid insomnia and depression represent a challenging group to treat. In depressed patients, insomnia is associated with an increased risk of suicide and sleep disturbances can persist long after successful depression treatment.[29,30] The anhedonia and low behavioral activation present in depressed patients can negatively affect their adherence to the behavioral recommendations of CBT-I.[31] Acupuncture that addresses comorbid depression may enhance motivation for and adherence to CBT-I. A 2017 systematic review and meta-analysis of 18 RCTs including 1,678 patients compared either combined acupuncture + medication (antidepressant, hypnotic, or both) or acupuncture alone against medication to treat depression-related insomnia.[32] Of the 10 studies that compared acupuncture against medication and reported PSQI scores, 7 showed acupuncture was more effective in reducing PSQI scores than medication, whereas 3 showed no difference between the groups.[32] Of the four studies that compared the combined acupuncture + medication against drug therapy alone, three found an advantage for the combined treatment over drug therapy in reducing PSQI scores, whereas one found no difference between groups.[32] These results suggest that acupuncture can be a promising adjunctive therapy to medication, and possibly CBT-I, for treating insomnia related to depression.

Menopausal symptoms

For many women, the transition to menopause is associated with significant sleep disturbance, and insomnia is one of the most reported symptoms in menopause.[33] Several factors associated with menopause have the potential to act as precipitating and perpetuating factors of insomnia, including vasomotor symptoms such as hot flash and night sweats, mood disorders, and shifts in hormonal activity.[34] Acupuncture has been investigated as a treatment option to address menopausal symptoms such as hot flashes in perimenopausal and postmenopausal women, as well as in women with breast cancer who experience early transition to menopause as a result of cancer treatment.[35] A 2017 systematic review and meta-analysis of 13 RCTs of acupuncture treatment in 844 patients with breast cancer found that acupuncture did not significantly reduce hot flash frequency or severity, but did significantly improve other menopause symptoms including paresthesia, depression, and joint pain.[36] Most recently, a 2021 systematic review and meta-analysis of 15 acupuncture trials involving 1,410 women with perimenopausal insomnia found

significantly reduced global PSQI scores (MD = −2.38) as well as improved menopausal symptoms in patients receiving acupuncture compared with controls.[37] Acupuncture was more effective in reducing menopausal symptoms, and had a higher clinical effectiveness rate for insomnia than hypnotic medications.[37] The available evidence supporting acupuncture to address menopausal symptoms in women with perimenopausal insomnia, menopausal insomnia, or breast cancer is encouraging. Acupuncture may be appropriate to explore as an adjunct treatment in patients for whom hormone-based therapies are contraindicated (ie, patients with breast cancer), and may be more effective in improving general distress associated with menopause symptoms than in reducing hot flash frequency and severity.

CHALLENGES WITH IMPLEMENTATION OF ACUPUNCTURE AS AN ADJUNCT TREATMENT

There remain several unanswered questions about whom CBT-I plus acupuncture would be most suited for and how these two treatments are best integrated for optimal effects. **Table 1** summarizes the unresolved patient and practical issues with using acupuncture as an adjunct to CBT-I.

Patient Characteristics Affecting Treatment Response

Patient characteristics have been shown to affect therapeutic response to different types of intervention. Acupuncture is a treatment with relatively large nonspecific treatment effects in contrast to

Table 1
Patient and practical issues with implementation of acupuncture as an adjunct to cognitive-behavioral therapy for insomnia

Patient Characteristics	Practical and Logistical Issues
1. Level of engagement required	1. Provider training requirements
2. Pretreatment sleep duration	2. Coordination of care
3. High objective/ subjective sleep discrepancy	3. Sequencing of treatments
4. Presence of comorbidities	4. Access and coverage
5. Treatment preference and expectancy	

CBT-I which directly targets theoretically supported mechanisms that contribute to the development and maintenance of insomnia. Therefore, it is reasonable to expect that patients who differ in certain demographic characteristics and life experience may react to acupuncture and CBT-I differently. Preliminary evidence suggests that gender, race, and education level may affect the magnitude of treatment response for both CBT-I and acupuncture.[28] Decisions about treatment should involve an informed discussion between patients and providers, and should take into account several factors, including (1) the level of active engagement that the treatment requires from the patient, (2) the specific characteristics of the patient's sleep disturbance (ie, whether it is characterized by short objective sleep duration, or high objective–subjective sleep discrepancy), (3) the presence or absence of physical and psychological comorbidities, and (4) the patient's treatment preference and expectancy. Understanding patient characteristics that influence treatment response is important to help patients and practitioners make informed, evidence-based decisions about care.

Level of engagement required

Before deciding on an insomnia treatment plan, patients and providers should clarify the level of engagement that the patient is able to commit to treatment. CBT-I requires significant engagement of the patient outside of treatment sessions to implement the components of sleep restriction and stimulus control, making adherence to its recommendations a key predictor of treatment response. Poor adherence to sleep restriction may be in part because of the counterintuitive recommendation to limit sleep, and inability to tolerate increased daytime sleepiness early in treatment, among other factors.[4] In contrast, acupuncture is viewed by the patient as a more passive intervention than CBT-I which requires less active effort and is more suited to insomnia related to physiologic factors, rather than insomnia related to psychological factors.[38] Rather than making significant alterations to their daily schedule, tracking their sleep, and physically leaving the bedroom during periods of sustained wakefulness, patients are simply required to attend a scheduled appointment with no obligations outside the treatment session itself. Patients who prefer a passive treatment or who are reluctant to make significant changes to their daily routine may perceive a better fit and find it easier to adhere to acupuncture. Supporting this, Garland and colleagues[28] found less attrition and more adherence for the acupuncture group

compared with the CBT-I group in a sample of cancer survivors. Practitioners should have an open and honest discussion with patients about the levels of effort involved with each treatment option, and the level of effort they are willing and able to commit to a therapy.

Pretreatment sleep duration

Another patient-related factor that may predict differential response to CBT-I and acupuncture is objective short sleep duration. Some researchers propose classification of insomnia subtypes based on objective sleep duration, with 6 h total sleep time as the cutoff separating insomnia with short sleep duration from insomnia with normal sleep duration.[39] Given that restricting time spent in bed is a core component of CBT-I, individuals with a habitual short sleep duration may be more reluctant to adhere to its recommendations, representing an implementation challenge in this patient group. Research supports that individuals with objective short sleep duration are less likely to adhere to or benefit from CBT-I compared with those with a normal sleep duration.[28,40,41] A not yet published secondary analysis of data from the RCT by Garland and colleagues[28] found greater improvements in insomnia severity immediately following CBT-I in individuals with normal sleep duration (ISI change score = -12.4) compared with short-sleepers (ISI change score = -10.0), which trended toward statistical significance ($P = .076$). In this analysis, 94% (29/31) of individuals with a normal sleep duration were classified as CBT-I responders, compared with only 68% (25/37) of short-sleepers, a difference which was statistically significant ($P = .014$). In the acupuncture group, no differences were found between short- and normal sleepers regarding ISI change score or proportion of treatment responders.[28] In this study cancer survivors with insomnia who underwent acupuncture treatment increased their total sleep time by 61.81 min at posttreatment, which was greater than the improvement observed in the CBT-I group (35.01 min).[28] This group difference was reduced, but still significant at a 3-month follow-up assessment.[28] Given the blunted treatment response to CBT-I and the risk of negative side effects to hypnotic medication such as dependence and cognitive impairment in patients with insomnia with short sleep duration, researchers are currently exploring acupuncture as a method of controlling physiologic hyperarousal, as the treatment has been shown to regulate HPA axis activity.[42]

Subjective–objective sleep discrepancy

Another group of patients who may respond differently to treatment are patients with a large difference between objective measures of sleep duration and their own subjective assessment. These patients underreport their sleep duration when compared with objective measurements obtained through actigraphy or polysomnography. In a prospective cohort study investigating the relationship between sleep discrepancy and CBT-I response, patients high in sleep discrepancy reported greater improvements in subjective total sleep time, sleep onset latency, and insomnia severity ratings following CBT-I treatment relative to patients with low sleep discrepancy.[43] There is some evidence that subjective–objective sleep discrepancy also influences response to acupuncture. Those with less objective–subjective sleep discrepancy were more likely to respond to placebo acupuncture than true acupuncture.[44,45] Responders to placebo acupuncture (defined by a minimum 8-point reduction in ISI scores at 1-week posttreatment) were characterized by higher insomnia severity ratings, higher sleep diary total sleep time and higher expectation toward acupuncture at baseline when compared with nonresponders, although only insomnia severity ratings were significant.[44] Responders to true acupuncture had a higher mean level of education and higher baseline insomnia severity ratings than nonresponders.[45] Individuals with greater subjective–objective sleep discrepancy may benefit more from acupuncture combined with training in sleep-wake discrimination, which can be included in the cognitive restructuring component of CBT-I when appropriate.

Presence of comorbidities
Another patient-related factor that can hinder response to insomnia treatment is the presence of psychiatric or physical comorbidities such as anxiety or chronic pain, which can exacerbate insomnia symptoms and impair both treatment adherence and response.[40] As reviewed above, CBT-I has shown effectiveness in improving the sleep of patients with comorbid insomnia, as well as small-to-moderate effects on comorbid symptoms, particularly in those with psychological rather than physical comorbidities.[8,9,31] Nonetheless, researchers continue to explore whether adjunct or alternative treatments such as acupuncture may confer additional benefit in improving sleep by addressing comorbid conditions. Patients who respond to acupuncture for insomnia typically report that it helped them sleep by lessening the burden of sleep-interfering comorbid conditions. Romero and colleagues[46] conducted posttreatment semi-structured interviews with cancer survivors randomized to the acupuncture arm of a clinical trial for insomnia treatment to determine patient characteristics that were related to acupuncture treatment response. Patients in this study reported that the alleviation of comorbid symptoms contributing to insomnia were strongly related to insomnia improvement. In contrast, when comorbidities such as hot flashes or pain were not sufficiently addressed by the treatment, it made it difficult for nonresponders to perceive improvements in sleep.[46]

Treatment preference and expectancy
Patient preference for a particular treatment may play a large role in determining critical factors to treatment response such as expectancy and adherence. A qualitative study investigating insomnia treatment preferences for CBT-I or acupuncture in cancer survivors found that patients tended to prefer the treatment they perceived as having a stronger evidence base, although whether the evidence was perceived to be greater for CBT-I or acupuncture varied between participants.[38] Patients who preferred acupuncture accepted its long history of use as evidence of its effectiveness, and believed that its use to treat ailments like pain and anxiety supported its use to treat insomnia. Those who preferred CBT-I felt that the treatment had strong empirical support, was scientifically driven, logical, and appropriate for insomnia treatment.[38] A high degree of treatment expectancy has been linked with both increased treatment adherence and improvement in subjective sleep indices.[40] Interestingly, those with lower sleep diary total sleep time are less likely to respond to placebo acupuncture, suggesting a limited role of expectancy in improving the sleep of these patients.[44] In a secondary analysis of an RCT in cancer survivors, patient expectancy for acupuncture, but not CBT-I, was associated with greater insomnia symptom reduction and treatment response (Xiaotong, unpublished data, January 2022). In the acupuncture group, patients with high expectancy achieved two times the treatment response rate at Week 8 than those with low expectancy (76% vs 38%); however, the treatment response rate was not associated with high or low expectancy (83% vs 70%) in the CBT-I group. For patients with high expectancy for acupuncture, both acupuncture and CBT-I provided an almost identical reduction in insomnia; therefore, the final treatment decision rests on availability of providers as well as patient preference (Xiaotong, unpublished data, January 2022). These results suggest that pretreatment preference and expectancy can be used to personalize insomnia management but further research is needed to explore how this affects in populations other than cancer and pain.

Practical and Logistical Issues Affecting Implementation

Delivery of acupuncture as an adjunct treatment to CBT-I requires consideration of several practical and logistical issues, including professional training requirements, access to and coverage for care, and sequencing of treatments.

Provider training requirements

The question of who will deliver acupuncture as an adjunct treatment to CBT-I is complicated, as the treatments are delivered by different classes of professionals, and access to both is somewhat scarce. CBT-I is typically delivered by a licensed psychologist or allied health professional, although there have been concerns that the number of available providers is far too small to meet the demand for behavior-based sleep interventions.[47] This scarcity is due in part to inadequate education and training to treat sleep disorders. In the United States and Canada, psychologists reported a median of 10 h of didactic training in sleep.[48] In fact, it is estimated that of the 167 US cities with a population greater than 150,000, 105 cities have no CBT-I providers.[47] The prevalence of CBT-I providers outside the United States is even more dire, but significant progress is being made to establish standards for training programs across Europe.[49] By contrast, acupuncture is typically delivered by (1) a licensed traditional acupuncturist or (2) medical doctors with additional acupuncture training.[50] For those who are not traditional acupuncture providers or physicians, the World Health Organization released acupuncture guidelines in 1999 noting that "basic training in acupuncture" might be defined as a minimum of 200 h recommended for physician practitioners.[50] The effect of this policy is that acupuncture may be easier to access than CBT-I, owing to a larger number of providers, although the training level of these providers may vary greatly. Although treatment protocols for insomnia have been developed in the context of research, it is unknown how much training acupuncturists receive in treating insomnia specifically.

Coordination of care

The difficulty of coordinating care between two providers who work in different settings raises the possibility of only one practitioner delivering the combined regimen. In this scenario, it may be more practical to instruct practitioners of acupuncture how to deliver components of CBT-I than for psychologists to integrate needling into their practice, as many acupuncturists already include elements of talk therapy into their sessions, and a psychologist would require at least several hundred additional hours of training in most areas before they were qualified to practice needling. Moreover, the behavioral components of CBT-I are manualized and relatively straightforward to understand. Acupuncturists would likely need training and supervision in cognitive therapy to implement the cognitive restructuring component of CBT-I. It is also important to acknowledge in acupuncture practice, the face-to face interaction often is brief and during the context of needle insertion or removal. As such what can be communicated verbally needs to be realistic to fit into the workflow of acupuncturists' practice. Research is needed to determine the efficacy and relative advantages and disadvantages of a combined treatment being delivered by one specialist.

Sequencing of treatments

The sequencing of treatments is another open question that has yet to be answered. It is possible that concurrent treatment with acupuncture and CBT-I would result in the most rapid sleep improvement, as acupuncture may help to increase total sleep time,[28] reduce discomfort from sleep-interfering physical symptoms, and its passive nature is unlikely to overwhelm patients committing to both treatments at once. However, this may be a more intensive treatment course and patients may not be able to commit to longer or more frequent sessions. There may be ways to creatively combine acupuncture with digital CBT-I which would eliminate the need for two skilled providers, but the feasibility and efficacy of this has yet to be evaluated. If not delivered concurrently, it is unknown which sequence of treatments would provide optimal outcomes, whether this would vary by individual, and what the most appropriate 'dose' would be.

Access and coverage

Also complicating matters is the question of cost and coverage. Most people receiving CBT-I or acupuncture in North America pay out of pocket. These treatments may be easier to access in places where they are covered by public health plans and/or private insurance payers but this remains the minority of places. Additional out of pocket costs for acupuncture as an adjunct treatment of insomnia, or vice versa, may be too large a burden for the relative benefit. Until we can address these practical and logistical issues, the feasibility and effectiveness of using acupuncture as an adjunct treatment with CBT-I will remain unknown.

SUMMARY AND RECOMMENDATIONS FOR FUTURE RESEARCH

In summary, the evidence to date supports the effectiveness of acupuncture to treat both insomnia disorder and improve symptoms associated with co-occurring conditions, including pain, depression, and hot flashes. True acupuncture outperforms both sham acupuncture and no treatment controls in reducing insomnia severity, suggesting the effects exceed that of treatment expectancy. Acupuncture is generally safer and more effective than medication in improving sleep quality. Although CBT-I may have a larger effect on insomnia severity, acupuncture produces clinically significant reductions in insomnia symptoms, and should not be overlooked as an adjunct treatment, especially in patients who prefer passive intervention, have short sleep duration, comorbid conditions, and more favorable attitudes and expectancy about acupuncture.

Future research is needed to address many of the above practical issues. Preliminary findings suggest some unique patient characteristics may affect response to CBT-I versus acupuncture. Machine learning techniques may be useful in determining how best to personalize treatment based on patient characteristics.[51] Prospective trials can evaluate whether precision delivery of interventions based on these factors can lead to better patient outcomes. Multiphase optimization strategies (MOST) can be used to develop and test efficient, effective delivery strategies for using acupuncture as an adjunct to CBT-I and help determine which components are needed to provide efficient and effective clinical care.[52] Subsequently, there may also be ways to use sequential multiple assignment randomized trial (SMART) or other adaptive designs to personalize and scale up/down treatment depending on patient response.[53] These lines of research can help ensure individuals with insomnia will receive the treatment that is most aligned with their preference and characteristics and most likely to produce clinically meaningful improvement.

CLINICS CARE POINTS

- While CBT-I is more effective in improving insomnia symptoms, evidence supports the effectiveness of acupuncture to bring clinically meaningful improvements in both insomnia and sleep interfering comorbid conditions such as pain, depression, or hot flashes.
- Acupuncture may address physical symptoms such as pain more effectively than CBT-I, making it an attractive treatment option for patients with sleep interfering physical comorbidities.
- Acupuncture carries lower risk for side effects or adverse events compared with sleep medications.
- Acupuncture treatment typically involves greater adherence and less attrition compared with CBT-I, likely due to its low level of required engagement.

DISCLOSURE

The authors have no commercial or financial conflicts of interest. Dr S.N. Garland is supported by an Emerging Scholar Award from the Canadian Cancer Society. Dr J.J. Mao is supported in part by National Institutes of Health, United States/National Cancer Institute Cancer Center grants (grant number P30 CA008748; 1 R01 CA240417-01A1).

REFERENCES

1. Qaseem A, Kansagara D, Forciea MA, et al. Management of chronic insomnia disorder in adults: a clinical practice guideline from the American College of Physicians. Ann Intern Med 2016;165(2):125–33.
2. Edinger JD, Arnedt JT, Bertisch SM, et al. Behavioral and psychological treatments for chronic insomnia disorder in adults: an American Academy of Sleep Medicine clinical practice guideline. J Clin Sleep Med 2021;17(2):255–62.
3. Mellor A, Hamill K, Jenkins MM, et al. Partner-assisted cognitive behavioural therapy for insomnia versus cognitive behavioural therapy for insomnia: a randomised controlled trial. Trials 2019;20(1):262.
4. Matthews EE, Arnedt JT, McCarthy MS, et al. Adherence to cognitive behavioral therapy for insomnia: a systematic review. Sleep Med Rev 2013;17(6):453–64.
5. Ong JC, Kuo TF, Manber R. Who is at risk for dropout from group cognitive-behavior therapy for insomnia? J Psychosom Res 2008;64(4):419–25.
6. Savard J, Ivers H, Savard MH, et al. Long-term effects of two formats of cognitive behavioral therapy for insomnia comorbid with breast cancer. Sleep 2016;39(4):813–23.
7. Arnedt JT, Cuddihy L, Swanson LM, et al. Randomized controlled trial of telephone-delivered cognitive behavioral therapy for chronic insomnia. Sleep 2013;36(3):353–62.
8. Carney CE, Edinger JD, Kuchibhatla M, et al. Cognitive behavioral insomnia therapy for those with insomnia and depression: a randomized controlled clinical trial. Sleep 2017;40(4). https://doi.org/10.1093/sleep/zsx019.

9. Wu JQ, Appleman ER, Salazar RD, et al. Cognitive Behavioral Therapy for Insomnia comorbid with psychiatric and medical conditions: a meta-analysis. JAMA Intern Med 2015;175(9):1461.

10. Taylor DJ, Mallory LJ, Lichstein KL, et al. Comorbidity of chronic insomnia with medical problems. Sleep 2007;30(2):213–8.

11. Khurshid KA. Comorbid insomnia and psychiatric disorders: an update. Innov Clin Neurosci 2018; 15(3–4):28–32.

12. Ostovar-Kermani T, Arnaud D, Almaguer A, et al. Painful sleep: insomnia in patients with chronic pain syndrome and its consequences. Folia Med (Plovdiv) 2020;62(4):645–54.

13. Cuijpers P, Cristea IA, Karyotaki E, et al. How effective are cognitive behavior therapies for major depression and anxiety disorders? A meta-analytic update of the evidence. World Psychiatry 2016; 15(3):245–58.

14. Zia FZ, Olaku O, Bao T, et al. The national cancer institute's conference on acupuncture for symptom management in oncology: state of the science, evidence, and research gaps. J Natl Cancer Inst Monogr 2017;2017(52). https://doi.org/10.1093/jncimonographs/lgx005.

15. Zhao K. Acupuncture for the treatment of insomnia. In: Int Rev Neurobiol111. Elsevier; 2013. p. 217–34.

16. Spence DW, Kayumov L, Chen A, et al. Acupuncture increases nocturnal melatonin secretion and reduces insomnia and anxiety: a preliminary report. J Neuropsychiatry Clin Neurosci 2004;16(1):19–28.

17. Kung Y, Yang C, Chiu J, et al. The relationship of subjective sleep quality and cardiac autonomic nervous system in postmenopausal women with insomnia under auricular acupressure. Menopause 2011;18(6). https://doi.org/10.1097/gme.0b013e318 20159c1. New York, NY.

18. Lee B, Shim I, Lee HJ, et al. Effects of acupuncture on chronic corticosterone-induced depression-like behavior and expression of neuropeptide Y in the rats. Neurosci Lett 2009;453(3):151–6.

19. Han JS. Acupuncture and endorphins. Neurosci Lett 2004;361(1–3):258–61.

20. Cao HJ, Yu ML, Wang LQ, et al. Acupuncture for primary insomnia: an updated systematic review of randomized controlled trials. J Altern Complement Med 2019;25(5):451–74.

21. Zhao FY, Fu QQ, Kennedy GA, et al. Can acupuncture improve objective sleep indices in patients with primary insomnia? a systematic review and meta-analysis. Sleep Med 2021;80:244–59.

22. Cheatle MD, Foster S, Pinkett A, et al. Assessing and managing sleep disturbance in patients with chronic pain. Anesthesiology Clin 2016;34(2):379–93.

23. Sivertsen B, Lallukka T, Petrie KJ, et al. Sleep and pain sensitivity in adults. Pain 2015;156(8):1433–9.

24. Yang M, Liou KT, Garland SN, et al. Acupuncture versus Cognitive Behavioral Therapy for pain among cancer survivors with insomnia: an exploratory analysis of a randomized clinical trial. npj Breast Cancer 2021;7(1):148.

25. Cherkin DC, Deyo RA, Sherman KJ, et al. Characteristics of visits to licensed acupuncturists, chiropractors, massage therapists, and naturopathic physicians. J Am Board Fam Pract 2002;15(6):463–72.

26. Vickers AJ, Vertosick EA, Lewith G, et al. Acupuncture for chronic pain: update of an individual patient data meta-analysis. J Pain 2018;19(5):455–74.

27. He Y, Guo X, May BH, et al. Clinical evidence for association of acupuncture and acupressure with improved cancer pain: a systematic review and meta-analysis. JAMA Oncol 2020;6(2):271–8.

28. Garland SN, Xie SX, DuHamel K, et al. Acupuncture versus Cognitive Behavioral Therapy for Insomnia in cancer survivors: a randomized clinical trial. J Natl Cancer Inst 2019;111(12):1323–31.

29. Carney CE, Segal ZV, Edinger JD, et al. A comparison of rates of residual insomnia symptoms following pharmacotherapy or cognitive-behavioral therapy for major depressive disorder. J Clin Psychiatry 2007;68(2):254–60.

30. Woznica AA, Carney CE, Kuo JR, et al. The insomnia and suicide link: toward an enhanced understanding of this relationship. Sleep Med Rev 2015;22:37–46.

31. Manber R, Bernert RA, Suh S, et al. CBT for insomnia in patients with high and low depressive symptom severity: adherence and clinical outcomes. J Clin Sleep Med 2011;7(6):645–52.

32. Dong B, Chen Z, Yin X, et al. The efficacy of acupuncture for treating depression-related insomnia compared with a control group: a systematic review and meta-analysis. Biomed Res Int 2017; 2017:9614810.

33. Drake CL, Kalmbach DA, Arnedt JT, et al. Treating chronic insomnia in postmenopausal women: a randomized clinical trial comparing cognitive-behavioral therapy for insomnia, sleep restriction therapy, and sleep hygiene education. Sleep 2019; 42(2). https://doi.org/10.1093/sleep/zsy217.

34. Proserpio P, Marra S, Campana C, et al. Insomnia and menopause: a narrative review on mechanisms and treatments. Climacteric 2020;23(6):539–49.

35. Harris PF, Remington PL, Trentham-Dietz A, et al. Prevalence and treatment of menopausal symptoms among breast cancer survivors. J Pain Symptom Manage 2002;23(6):501–9.

36. Chien TJ, Hsu CH, Liu CY, et al. Effect of acupuncture on hot flush and menopause symptoms in breast cancer- a systematic review and meta-analysis. PLoS One 2017;12(8):e0180918.

37. Zhao FY, Fu QQ, Kennedy GA, et al. Comparative utility of acupuncture and western medication in

the management of perimenopausal insomnia: a systematic review and meta-analysis. Evid Based Complement Alternat Med 2021;2021:5566742. https://doi.org/10.1155/2021/5566742. eCollection 2021.

38. Garland SN, Eriksen W, Song S, et al. Factors that shape preference for acupuncture or cognitive behavioral therapy for the treatment of insomnia in cancer patients. Support Care Cancer 2018;26(7): 2407–15.

39. Vgontzas AN, Fernandez-Mendoza J, Liao D, et al. Insomnia with objective short sleep duration: the most biologically severe phenotype of the disorder. Sleep Med Rev 2013;17(4):241–54.

40. Cho JH, Kremer S, Young J. Who to refer to a behavioral insomnia clinic? - recommendations based on treatment rationale and response prediction. Curr Sleep Med Rep 2021;17:1–8.

41. Bathgate CJ, Edinger JD, Krystal AD. Insomnia patients with objective short sleep duration have a blunted response to Cognitive Behavioral Therapy for Insomnia. Sleep 2017;40(1):zsw012.

42. Wang C, Yang WJ, Yu XT, et al. Acupuncture for insomnia with short sleep duration: protocol for a randomised controlled trial. BMJ Open 2020;10(3): e033731.

43. Ahn JS, Bang YR, Jeon HJ, et al. Effects of subjective-objective sleep discrepancy on the response to cognitive behavior therapy for insomnia. J Psychosom Res 2021;152:110682.

44. Yeung WF, Chung KF, Yu BYM, et al. Response to placebo acupuncture in insomnia: a secondary analysis of three randomized controlled trials. Sleep Med 2015;16(11):1372–6.

45. Yeung WF, Chung KF, Yu YMB, et al. What predicts a positive response to acupuncture? a secondary analysis of three randomised controlled trials of insomnia. Acupunct Med 2017;35(1):24–9.

46. Romero SAD, Jiang E, Bussell J, et al. What makes one respond to acupuncture for insomnia? Perspectives of cancer survivors. Palliat Support Care 2020; 18(3):301–6.

47. Thomas A, Grandner M, Nowakowski S, et al. Where are the behavioral sleep medicine providers and where are they needed? A geographic assessment. Behav Sleep Med 2016;14(6):687–98.

48. Zhou ES, Mazzenga M, Gordillo ML, et al. Sleep education and training among practicing clinical psychologists in the United States and Canada. Behav Sleep Med 2021;19(6):744–53.

49. Baglioni C, Altena E, Bjorvatn B, et al. The European Academy for cognitive behavioural therapy for insomnia: an initiative of the European insomnia network to promote implementation and dissemination of treatment. J Sleep Res 2020;29(2):e12967.

50. Ijaz N, Boon H. Evaluating the international standards gap for the use of acupuncture needles by physiotherapists and chiropractors: a policy analysis. PLoS One 2019;14(12):e0226601.

51. Hilbert K, Kunas SL, Lueken U, et al. Predicting cognitive behavioral therapy outcome in the outpatient sector based on clinical routine data: a machine learning approach. Behav Res Ther 2020; 124:103530.

52. Collins LM, Murphy SA, Strecher V. The multiphase optimization strategy (MOST) and the sequential multiple assignment randomized trial (SMART): new methods for more potent eHealth interventions. Am J Prev Med 2007;32(5 Suppl):S112–8.

53. Ghosh P, Nahum-Shani I, Spring B, et al. Noninferiority and equivalence tests in sequential, multiple assignment, randomized trials (SMARTs). Psychol Methods 2020;25(2):182–205.